AIDS: A SELF-CARE MANUAL

▲ AIDS PROJECT LOS ANGELES

EDITORS

BettyClare Moffatt, M.A.

Judith Spiegel, M.P.H.

Steve Parrish

Michael Helquist

Third Edition Copyright 1989

AIDS: A Self-Care Manual
by AIDS Project Los Angeles

Edited by:
BettyClare Moffatt, M.A.
Judy Spiegel, M.P.H.
Steve Parrish
Michael Helquist

First Edition Copyright 1987 by AIDS Project Los Angeles
Cover Design Copyright 1987

Published by:
IBS Press
744 Pier Avenue
Santa Monica, CA 90405
(213)450-6485

In Cooperation with:
AIDS Project Los Angeles
6721 Romaine Street
West Hollywood, CA 90038
(213)962-1600

Design and type composition by:
Highpoint Type & Graphics, Inc.

Printed in the U.S.A.
First printing: June, 1987
Second printing: June, 1988
Third printing: August, 1989

Library of Congress Catalog Card Number 89-80892
ISBN 1-877880-00-0

Note: Portions of this book originally appeared under the title *Living with AIDS: A Self-Care Manual,* Copyright 1984 by AIDS Project Los Angeles.

Dedication

Since the beginning of the AIDS epidemic, people with AIDS, ARC, and HIV infection have provided ongoing inspiration and motivation to those who work to see the day when AIDS is prevented throughout the world. Their courage, sense of humor, and determination offer an example about living well in the light of a personal and national crisis. Their strength reveals the power of human compassion and commitment. Our debt to them is ongoing; history will record their contribution.

This guide is dedicated to those who live with AIDS today and to those whom we have lost in the battle against this illness. They have enriched our lives and nourished our daily efforts; our memories of them will enhance our future.

Judith Spiegel, MPH
AIDS Project Los Angeles

This third edition of *AIDS: A Self-Care Manual* is dedicated to the loving memory of my son Michael Welsch, who died of AIDS on July 14, 1986, and to all the families everywhere who are touched and transformed by the AIDS crisis.

BettyClare Moffatt
President
IBS Press

Acknowledgments

Our sincere thanks to the many health-care workers, volunteers, and people with HIV infection for their donated time and energy to the production of this guide. We would also like to thank those authors and organizations that allowed us to reprint their articles and brochures, especially the AIDS Health Project in San Francisco, the San Francisco AIDS Foundation, and Southern California CARES. A complete list of contributors can be found at the back of this volume.

About AIDS Project Los Angeles

AIDS Project Los Angeles (APLA) is a non-profit public health organization dedicated to providing vital support to people with AIDS and AIDS-related illnesses and education to the general community.

The purpose of AIDS Project Los Angeles is:

- to support and maintain the best possible quality of life for persons in Los Angeles County with AIDS and AIDS-related illnesses, and their loved ones, by providing and promoting publicly and privately funded vital human services for them;

- to reduce the overall incidence of human immunodeficiency virus (HIV) infection by providing risk-reduction education and information for persons primarily affected by and at risk for AIDS, and the general public;

- to reduce the levels of fear and discrimination directed toward persons affected by AIDS, and to enhance and preserve the dignity and self-respect of those persons, by providing and promoting critically needed education to the public, health-care providers, educators, business and religious leaders, the media, public officials, and other opinion leaders; and

- to ensure the ongoing support for all of these services by involving, educating, and cooperating with a wide range of organizations and individuals in AIDS-related service provision, and by supporting efforts at all levels of the public and private sectors to secure adequate development and finance of AIDS research, education, and human service programs.

A Note from the Publisher

IBS Press is honored to present this Third Edition of *AIDS: A Self-Care Manual* with the cooperation of AIDS Project Los Angeles. Since the initial publication of *AIDS: A Self-Care Manual,* the book has reached over 50,000 people and AIDS organizations.

This Third Edition contains all-new, updated appendixes listing AIDS-related organizations and helpful books, tapes and periodicals.

Medical research in the field of AIDS is constantly advancing. The situation changes daily, and new hope for extended life-spans is on the horizon. Because both traditional and alternative treatments for AIDS are still in flux, *AIDS: A Self-Care Manual* presents only the basic medical information and self-care procedures needed by all PWAs. Please contact your doctor or local AIDS agency for additional information.

This Guide Is for You, If...

- you are worried about possibly being exposed to AIDS or HIV due to past sexual contacts or needle-sharing, intravenous drug use;

- you are wondering whether to be tested for the AIDS antibody to determine whether you have been exposed to the AIDS virus;

- you have received a positive or negative AIDS antibody result and want to know exactly what this means for you;

- you want to be sure you are up-to-date in your understanding of how to reduce your risk for coming into contact with the AIDS virus;

- your son or daughter, brother or sister has just been diagnosed with AIDS, ARC, or an HIV infection;

- you want to know how AIDS affects women, what the risks are to women, whether to become pregnant or not, and how to protect yourself;

- you have heard that people of color also get AIDS and you want to know how to reduce your risk of exposure;

- you are worried that a classmate of your child might have AIDS and wonder whether your child is at risk;

- you are a parent and want help talking with your children about the AIDS epidemic;

- you believe someone in your office may be infected with the AIDS virus and you want to know if it is safe to share the office with that person;

- you want to know how to help your best friend, colleague, spouse, or partner who has been diagnosed with AIDS or ARC or who has discovered that he or she has been exposed to the AIDS virus;

- you are caring for someone with AIDS at home and you want to protect yourself from infection while allowing the individual the highest quality of life possible;

- you are a parent or other family member of someone with the AIDS virus and you need help coping with the emotional aspects of caring for your loved one with AIDS;

- you have been diagnosed with AIDS or ARC and want to maintain the best health you can, finding the ways you can help your immune system fight the infection;

- you want to know about medical treatments and possible side effects of available treatments;

- you want more information about alternative forms of medical care and need help choosing which ones are right for you;

- you need help obtaining benefits and government financial assistance or want help determining what insurance coverage you now have or want to obtain;

- you feel drawn to explore the spiritual dimensions of your circumstances and your present life and want to know what others think about the role of spirituality and healing within the context of AIDS;

- you want to help stop the spread of AIDS in your community, recognizing that being well-informed will help you educate others to reduce their risk without becoming unreasonably scared of AIDS.

So many of us are affected by the AIDS epidemic that, in a sense, we all live with AIDS in our midst. This health crisis challenges us as individuals and as a society to come together to help one another, to be informed, and to stop the spread of AIDS.

One of the most important things to know about AIDS is that it *is* preventable. No one else need be infected by the AIDS virus; but to stop AIDS in its tracks, we must educate ourselves and those individuals we care about. This guide provides the information for you to become an active and caring member in the team effort to block AIDS and to treat those infected with the virus with understanding and compassion.

Table of Contents

How to Use This Manual

This manual is comprehensive in its coverage of many of the concerns and needs of people exposed to the AIDS virus, diagnosed with AIDS symptoms, worried about AIDS, and grieving for those who have been diagnosed with the disease. This information is presented to help concerned individuals learn all they can about the AIDS epidemic. We believe that this book can help you better care for yourself and your loved ones, feel more in control of your own life, and help you work with health care providers to obtain the best care possible.

Section One, AIDS: AN OVERVIEW, presents current basic information on AIDS, as well as current facts and fictions about AIDS.

Comprehensive medical information, intended primarily for health-care providers, is covered in greater detail in Section Three, A MEDICAL PER-SPECTIVE; Section Four, TREATMENT: A THERAPEUTIC PERSPEC-TIVE; and in the symptom management portion of Section Six, A SELF-CARE PERSPECTIVE. So a reader concerned with the medical management of AIDS would look in Sections Three, Four, and Six, although there is, of course, con-siderable overlapping information in other sections of this book.

Section Two, A SOCIO-PSYCHOLOGICAL PERSPECTIVE, deals with various aspects of the needs of a person with AIDS, the family, the friends, the workplace, the social implications of youth and children at risk, and finally, the impact of AIDS seen in the light of a terminal illness. Here the concerns are more personal, more meaningful. It is suggested that everyone concerned with the AIDS crisis would especially benefit from Section Two, A SOCIO-PSYCHOLOGICAL PERSPECTIVE, as well as Section Nine, A HEALING PERSPECTIVE.

In addition to the medical data, Section Three offers useful general infor-mation about every type of AIDS-related illness, including AIDS infections and malignancies, ARC, Hemophilia, and an integrated power approach to the AIDS health problem.

Section Four, TREATMENT: A THERAPEUTIC PERSPECTIVE, offers alternative approaches to AIDS wellness, along with more information on the medical aspects of AIDS.

Section Five, PREVENTION: A SOCIO-SEXUAL PERSPECTIVE, car-ries the following disclaimer, *"Warning: Sexually explicit material. NOT read-ing this can be dangerous to your health."* This section should be read by *every* sexually active man and woman, whether heterosexual, bisexual, or homosexual. Presented in clinical, sexually explicit language, the information can quite possibly save your life. This section is a valuable, life-enhancing, practical tool for all sexually active persons.

Section Six, A SELF-CARE PERSPECTIVE, offers practical and useful home care guidelines, as well as nutrition, hygiene, dental care, and symptom management. Care-givers, including family members, will find this section especially helpful, as will the person with AIDS.

Section Seven, A PRACTICAL PERSPECTIVE, helps the person with AIDS to take care of business. It covers social services, benefits, and the practical aspects of making a will and power of attorney. Of special interest is a comprehensive guide to health, disability, and life insurance in "Understanding Your Insurance Policies." Every person with AIDS can benefit greatly from reading and applying the ideas presented in this section.

Section Eight, A SPIRITUAL PERSPECTIVE, written by an esteemed team of ministers from various denominations, offers a thoughtful assessment of spiritual issues and needs. This section is *not* just for the clergy. On the contrary, the spiritual awakening that often accompanies a life-threatening illness spills over into the lives of everyone connected with the AIDS patient.

Section Nine, A HEALING PERSPECTIVE, offers life enhancing acceptance and love in the very face of death with "Experiencing the Powers of Healing," a moving account of a friend's search for healing in the face of death; "A Healing Meditation"; and finally, a legacy of love from a son to his mother as they go through the final days of his life together.

Section Ten, SELF-CARE RESOURCES, offers a wealth of useful information through the glossary of AIDS-related terms, as well as the two appendices: one listing AIDS-related organizations and hotlines; the other listing current helpful books, pamphlets, and tapes related to AIDS. Following the Index are several self-help forms and charts for use by persons with AIDS and by care-givers.

Suggested Reading

It is not necessary to read through this book in one sitting, and some sections may not be relevant to your own interests and concerns. We suggest that you briefly look through each section to become familiar with what is available, and then focus on those sections that most directly answer your questions. We do recommend again that *all* readers look through the segment on AIDS prevention and specific risk reduction in Section Five, PREVENTION: A SOCIO-SEXUAL PERSPECTIVE. This information can help save your life and the lives of those you care about.

For further AIDS-related information, consult with your local AIDS organization and your physician or other health-care provider. Most importantly, remember that you are not alone. All people have some concerns about AIDS. Know that people are here to help you. This book, *AIDS: A Self-Care Manual*, is here to help you too.

Section One

AIDS: An Overview

Anyone, regardless of gender, race, age, or sexual orientation could contract or transmit AIDS. ☑ *TRUE* ☐ *FALSE*

There is little an individual can do to help. ☐ *TRUE* ☑ *FALSE*

"Fact vs. Fiction"

AIDS: An Overview
Fact vs. Fiction
AIDS Risk in Public Places

AIDS: An Overview

What is AIDS?

Aquired immune deficiency syndrome (AIDS) is an impairment of the body's immune system which occurs in previously healthy individuals. While this impairment affects only a portion of the immune system, affected individuals are left vulnerable to illnesses which might not otherwise occur. These illnesses include opportunistic infections and rare cancers.

What Are Opportunistic Infections?

Opportunistic infections are caused by organisms commonly found in the environment which are resisted by the normal immune system. When the immune system is not functioning properly, these organisms seize the "opportunity" to infect the body.

What Are the Opportunistic Infections Associated with AIDS?

Many opportunistic infections are associated with AIDS. The most common include pneumocystis carinii pneumonia (PCP); chronic, persistent cytomegalovirus (CMV); severe, prolonged candidiasis (yeast infections); unusually extensive herpes of prolonged duration; toxoplasmosis; and an unusual form of tuberculosis.

What About Kaposi's Sarcoma?

Kaposi's sarcoma (KS), an otherwise rare form of cancer, has frequently been reported in many cases of AIDS and is considered to be an "opportunistic" cancer. Many people with AIDS do not have and may never develop Kaposi's sarcoma.

Is Immune Suppression the Same as AIDS?

All individuals who have AIDS are immune suppressed; however, the reverse is not always true. Many infections, such as cytomegalovirus, hepatitis, infectious mononucleosis, and others, cause temporary periods of immune suppression, but do not necessarily indicate AIDS and are not usually considered opportunistic.

What Causes AIDS?

AIDS is caused by a virus—now called HIV (human immunodeficiency virus)—which breaks down the body's immune system. The AIDS virus begins by attacking the body's T-cells, which are normally responsible for recognizing infections and alerting the immune system to begin producing antibodies. When the AIDS virus puts T-cells out of operation, the immune system cannot respond properly to serious illnesses.

What Are the Symptoms of AIDS?

Many of the AIDS symptoms are subtle and may only indicate simple, everyday ailments; therefore, you should be alerted but not alarmed if you have one or more of the following symptoms:

- weight loss of more than ten pounds during a period of less than two months that is not related to diet or increased activity;

- prolonged loss of appetite;

- unexplained, persistent or recurrent fevers, shaking chills, or night sweats;

- swollen glands (lymph nodes found in the neck, armpits, and groin) which persist and are unexplained by other illness;

- severe and prolonged fatigue that is not transient or explained by physical activity, substance abuse, or a psychological disorder;

- persistent and unexplained diarrhea or bloody stools;

- a persistent, whitish coating (or spotting) on the tongue or in the throat which may be accompanied by soreness or difficulty in swallowing;

- a heavy, persistent, dry cough that is not due to smoking and has lasted too long to be explained by a cold or flu;

- unexplained bleeding from any orifice.

Kaposi's sarcoma patients may have any of the above symptoms and/or might develop slowly enlarging purplish or discolored nodules, plaques, lumps, or other new growths on top of or beneath the skin or on mucous membranes (inside the mouth, nasal passages, anus, or underneath the eyelids). These lesions do not disappear and may get larger and cannot be explained as bruises, blood blisters, insect bites, or pimples.

What Should I Do If I Have Any of These Symptoms?

It must be emphasized that each of these symptoms may appear in diseases that are not caused by or associated with AIDS. The persistence of one or more of these symptoms should be discussed with a health-care provider who is familiar with AIDS.

Can AIDS Be Treated?

While there is no known cure for AIDS at this time, some of the accompanying infections and cancers can be treated. Advances in medical treatment have allowed some people with AIDS to live several years.

Am I at Risk?

Anyone who engages in high-risk activities with people who have been infected can contract the virus which causes AIDS. "High-risk activities" usually means intimate sexual contact or sharing intravenous drugs. The AIDS virus has infected people of all ages, races, and social groups.

Many people who have contracted the AIDS virus do not ever experience any symptoms and may never develop AIDS. The AIDS virus can remain in the body for six years or more, possibly as much as ten years, before symptoms appear.

Should I Avoid People with AIDS?

Being a friend won't give you AIDS. It *cannot* be spread through casual contact or through the air. That means working and attending school or social events with people who have AIDS is very safe. You can even hold someone's hand or give them a hug without worrying about contracting the AIDS virus.

Before long you will probably know someone with AIDS. It may happen to a friend, a family member, or a person you don't know very well. Just like you, people with AIDS need a lot of love and support. Many of them have been deserted by their families. Some have even lost their jobs or their homes. It doesn't take much to help someone with AIDS. All you have to do is be a friend.

How Can I Help?

AIDS and its related problems and issues are serious matters which affect the entire population. Many community-supported groups and individuals are united together in the fight against AIDS.

Talk to your friends and loved ones about AIDS. Make sure they know how AIDS is and is not transmitted. You can help stop the spread of AIDS today. Once you have the facts, it's simple. If you take responsibility for your own life you won't have to worry about anyone giving you AIDS. Just make the choices that will keep you alive and healthy.

Fact vs. Fiction

Ten Things You Should Know About AIDS

1. Little is actually known about AIDS.   ☐ True   ☑ False

We know that AIDS is caused by a virus called HIV (human immunodeficiency virus) that attacks and destroys the immune system and leaves the body vulnerable to a variety of life-threatening illnesses including rare types of skin cancer, pneumonia, meningitis, and dementia (mental illness). We also know how it is and isn't spread and how to protect ourselves from the disease.

What we don't know includes whether or not cofactors such as alcohol or drug abuse, poor nutrition, stress, or other illnesses play a role in the development of the disease; how long its incubation period lasts (although it has been proven to be as long as five to eight years, possibly up to ten); and what the long-term effects of infection are for people who have been exposed to the AIDS virus, but do not yet display any of its symptoms or associated life-threatening illnesses.

Reprinted from the brochure, "Fact vs. Fiction," published by the San Francisco AIDS Foundation.

2. Anyone, regardless of gender, race, age, or sexual orientation could contract or transmit AIDS. ☑ True   ☐ False

While over 70 percent of the AIDS patients in this country at the present time are gay, the numbers are changing daily as the disease also strikes heterosexuals, intravenous drug users, hemophiliacs, and their respective sex partners. In Africa, where over 50 percent of the population in some countries have been exposed to the AIDS virus, AIDS strikes primarily heterosexuals.

3. AIDS can be spread through casual contact. ☐ True   ☑ False

AIDS is transmitted only through clearly identifiable sexual activities and by blood to blood contact. According to Dr. James Curran, director of AIDS Activities for the Centers for Disease Control, "No evidence supports AIDS transmission by the airborne route, by objects handled by people with AIDS, or by contaminated environmental surfaces. There is also no evidence that saliva, sweat, or tears have transmitted the AIDS virus."

4. There is no simple test to diagnose AIDS. ☑ True   ☐ False

At the present time, AIDS can only be diagnosed by the existence of a life-threatening illness that would not otherwise be found in a person with a fully functioning immune system. There is, however, the AIDS antibody test, used primarily to screen the nation's blood supply, which can detect the presence of the AIDS antibody in the blood. The test does have an error factor of less than three percent.

5. There is a vaccine against AIDS. ☐ True   ☑ False

At this time, there is no vaccine that will make a person immune to AIDS. Understanding how the AIDS virus is spread and learning how to prevent its transmission are currently the only ways to slow the epidemic.

6. AIDS cannot be prevented. ☐ True   ☑ False

To avoid contracting or transmitting AIDS follow the same precautionary steps as with other sexually transmitted diseases—do not allow semen, blood, urine, feces, or vaginal secretions to enter the body. Use condoms for all types of sexual intercourse. Avoid other forms of blood-to-blood contact including the sharing of hypodermic needles, razors, and toothbrushes.

7. There is a high risk of acquiring AIDS from a blood transfusion.
☐ True   ☑ False

The nation's blood supply is now screened for HIV contamination and is considered to be safe.

8. The general public should not be concerned about AIDS.
☐ True   ☑ False

Already, over 10,000 Americans have been killed by this nearly always fatal disease. As of April 1987, 34,513 cases of AIDS have been reported. The number of people suffering from AIDS is expected to double every year, with increasing percentages of heterosexuals and others not now in the high-risk groups.

The economic and social impact of AIDS is staggering. Health-care costs average over $130,000 for each AIDS patient. Insurance premiums are rising in response to the AIDS crisis. In the workplace, co-workers with valuable skills and contributions to make are gone. Loved ones are lost. And a wave of hysteria, termed "AFRAIDS" by one national publication, threatens the civil rights and well-being of literally tens of millions of Americans—including many beyond the high-risk groups.

9. No end to this health crisis is in sight.   ☐ True   ☑ False

While there is currently no treatment or cure for people with AIDS, federal and private agencies are increasingly devoting more time and funding to AIDS research. And with increased public awareness about AIDS—its cause and transmission—the spread of the disease can be controlled.

Public education and social service programs like those of the San Francisco AIDS Foundation and AIDS Project Los Angeles also offer hope, tangible support, and desperately needed services.

10. There is little an individual can do to help   ☐ True   ☑ False

Being informed about AIDS is absolutely vital if the disease and the wave of hysteria accompanying it are to be controlled. It is also critical that we offer the same social and emotional support to AIDS patients as we would to anyone with a life-threatening illness.

AIDS Risk in Public Places

So, you've heard that terrible tale about AIDS—acquired immune deficiency syndrome. What do you really know about it? Or, more importantly, how much don't you know?

First of all, AIDS is NOT an easy thing to "catch." In fact, it's darned difficult. You really have to work at it. Since 1981, our public health experience with AIDS has shown that those people coming down with AIDS remain in the same basic groups year after year. Those groups of individuals do *not* include health-care workers caring for people with AIDS, nor do they include family members, friends, or co-workers who have only casual day-to-day contact. The AIDS virus does *not* travel through the air or pass through clothing. To catch it you must have sex or exchange blood (or other intimate body fluids) with a member of a high-risk group.

High-risk groups are where we most often see AIDS diagnosed. They include:

- Gay and bisexual men

- Intravenous drug users

- Hemophiliacs

- Blood transfusion recipients

- Sexual partners of the above groups

These groups most likely contracted AIDS through:
- —intimate sexual contact
- —sharing contaminated needles
- —using medical products made from blood
- —infected blood

Remember: Just because someone you know may be a "member" of a high-risk group does *not* mean that that person has AIDS, will come down with AIDS, or can spread the disease. As long as you don't have sexual contact or share blood products with this person, you are *not* at risk.

You can take healthy precautions to protect yourself and others. In fact, more often than not, you simply need to use those good old-fashioned daily rules that mother taught.

Personal Contact

The AIDS virus is not carried on clothing or in the air, so a pat on the back or a hug does not make you an endangered species. You can safely shake hands without rubber gloves with someone who has AIDS. People who give an occasional hug or touch (especially family members) are *not* at risk for coming down with AIDS. And in fact, it helps everyone concerned to maintain the same everyday relationships and behavior they have always had. That way no one will feel bad about ignoring or deserting a friend, and that friend with AIDS won't feel like an outcast.

The Bathroom

These simple rules are important to follow:

1) Always wash your hands after using the restroom to protect others and yourself.

2) Clean restroom facilities with household bleach diluted in water.

3) Whenever possible, wear rubber gloves to clean restroom facilities (this protects you from many germs and organisms).

It shouldn't be difficult to follow these rules as most of us were brought up believing the bathroom to be overflowing with germs. However, remember learning that all those "social diseases" are *not* spread by toilet seats and doorknobs? Well, neither is AIDS. People with AIDS can *safely* use the same restroom facilities as the general public. And, follow those signs in public restrooms that say WASH YOUR HANDS! (LAVE SUS MANOS!) Do it! This is a good safety measure for everyone. It rinses away germs that you contact (including your own), and protects you and the people around you.

Food and Drink

Caffeine and calories have lots of side effects (the jitters, weight problems, etc.), but AIDS is *not* one of them. Using the water cooler after someone with AIDS, sharing a pot of coffee, and eating in the same lunch room may be a way to spread gossip, but not AIDS.

As long as you have routine health practices, like washing your hands before eating or handling food, and as long as the person who prepares your food does the same, you are taking reasonable protective measures. Washing hands is the key to preventing lots of diseases, not just AIDS. If you do not use disposable eating utensils simply wash them in hot soapy water.

Cover your mouth when you sneeze or cough. This protects you and those around you from the common cold, and that's good. But AIDS is *not* spread through the air. Saliva doesn't seem to be an easy way to spread AIDS either. If it were a common way of getting AIDS, we would see far more cases—particularly in families of people with AIDS.

AIDS and the Workplace

If you're worried about where that pen has been, you need not. Office equipment and utensils do *not* spread AIDS. Unless tools have direct contact with blood (like medical equipment, razors, and sharp-edged instruments), there's no need to take unusual precautions in sharing them.

If you are concerned about re-using coffee cups, eating utensils, or equipment which might have had blood contact, here are a few hints:

1) Wash all re-usable eating utensils (including plates and cups) in *hot* soapy water.

2) Clean tools and counters with alcohol or household bleach. (Bleach can be diluted by adding nine parts water to one part bleach.)

3) Clean any blood spills or vomit with diluted household bleach. Dispose of paper towels in the waste can; cloth towels and rags should be washed in *hot* water.

4) Whenever possible, wear rubber gloves to clean spills that involve body fluids; and

5) Always wash your hands after contact with blood or other body fluids.

Blood. If you work in a job where there are likely to be accidents from time to time leading to bleeding, then here is a helpful hint: Those of you who are barbers, hairdressers, glass cutters, drafters, construction workers, you know that from time to time you cut or puncture yourselves. Slow down and use the normal daily precautions you would to avoid accidents. But, just in case accidents happen, follow the measures below:

1) Don't share equipment which has blood contact, or

2) Be sure to wash/sterilize contaminated equipment with alcohol or household bleach that is diluted in water. This is especially true of tools such as razors used by barbers.

3) Clean wounds thoroughly and cover them with a bandage to avoid further blood contact.

4) Clean spills with household bleach diluted in water.

5) Whenever possible, wear rubber gloves to clean.

6) Always wash your hands after contact with blood or other body fluids—no matter who is involved in the incident.

If you are concerned about the accident or wound, talk to your company or private doctor.

Conclusion

So, now you've heard the less than terrible truth about AIDS. Don't let your fears about AIDS imprison you or cause you to become strangers to your co-workers. AIDS can be a devastating life-threatening illness for those who have it, but it is *not* a danger to those who have only casual contact with people with AIDS.

If you are worried about AIDS, use the precautions presented here. Don't hesitate to get more information from your doctor, county health department, or AIDS Hotline. You can be the key to your own healthy peace of mind, and a support for those around you.

Section Two

A Socio-Psychological Perspective

I don't feel like a patient—passive, fearful, and immobolized. Rather, I am an active participant in the fight for my health, working with the doctors, molding my recovery, acknowledging my fears, and communicating as best I can.

"From the Heart: The Family's Response"

Meeting Psychological Needs in the AIDS Crisis

Stephen F. Morin, Ph.D.; Alan K. Malyon, Ph.D.;
David Epstein, Ph.D.; Allan Pinka, Ph.D.;
Kenneth A. Charles; Walter F. Batchelor

AIDS has a strong effect on all who come into contact with it. Whether you are the diagnosed person, a family member, a friend, or a care provider, you cannot help but be touched by the widespread implications of this disease. To many people working to stop the spread of AIDS, it is becoming increasingly clear that AIDS is as much a mental health crisis as it is a medical crisis. As a result, many individuals have begun to seek counseling and support for psychological burdens related to AIDS.

Spouses and lovers of persons with AIDS may have their own needs for psychological care. They may fear for their own health and they may be concerned about the amount of stress that results from caring for their diagnosed partner. Knowing that one has shared the most intimate contact with someone who is dying of a contagious disease can be shattering. Spouses and lovers are almost certain to face many of the same stressful situations along with those diagnosed as they help with daily tasks throughout the duration of their partner's illness. When individuals are diagnosed with AIDS, their family and friends are faced with a series of distressing issues. Spouses and friends who are also at high risk for AIDS may be particularly vulnerable because they can readily identify with those diagnosed. Indeed, friends and family often overidentify and act as if *they* have just been diagnosed. Other reactions might include awkwardness in discussing the illness, and problems in working through fears they have regarding contagion. Some of these people may want to be supportive but do not know how to provide that emotional support.

For many, the diagnosis of a friend leads to difficult reappraisals and evaluations of their own lifestyle with a resulting desire to learn new behavior for themselves. Learning for the first time that a friend or family member is gay (or an IV-drug user) can cause additional stress, making it difficult to cope with an already trying and complicated situation. For some, a diagnosis of AIDS becomes an automatic identifier for their being gay. Families that do not accept the homosexual orientation of an individual may find it particularly difficult to be supportive for the duration of the AIDS experience. Furthermore, the social stigma associated with the diagnosis involves a presumption, and sometimes a judgment, about an individual's lifestyle; there may be a fear—on the part of those diagnosed or for the family—of being "found out" by the general community.

Issues of bereavement may also be difficult for both friends and family. Since most persons with AIDS are fairly young, their partners, friends, and family may not be as equipped to deal with the issues of death and dying at an early age. There may also be a sense of injustice because of the "untimeliness" or "undeserved" nature of the illness.

The psychosocial needs of the person with AIDS are similar to those of the cancer patient. Almost always, the human response to a life-threatening illness is profound stress and despair. The primary aim of psychotherapeutic intervention (seeing a counselor or therapist) is to enhance a person's coping abilities and to provide emotional support. Such counseling can often help the diagnosed individual cope better with the many issues that occur with AIDS and ARC. In addition, family members and friends can provide emotional support and assistance.

The person diagnosed with AIDS, ARC, or HIV infection, as well as spouse, lover, family, and friends, may want to pursue different means of reducing the stress of the experience. Such techniques as relaxation training, biofeedback, and hypnosis may be helpful and improve the quality of living during these difficult times. Several of these techniques are discussed in greater detail in Section Four under "Alternative Treatments."

Sexuality

Many people infected with the AIDS virus will need help in adapting their sexual activities to their new status. The bottom line for all who have been exposed, as well as for those who want to avoid exposure to the AIDS virus, is to avoid the exchange of bodily fluids, such as blood and semen. (See Section Five, PREVENTION: A SOCIO-SEXUAL PERSPECTIVE.)

Individuals may need help in setting and maintaining sexual limits for themselves. They may also need help from counselors and educators to develop assertiveness and the social skills necessary to be able to negotiate these sexual limits with their partners. Some people use sex to reduce anxiety. For them, the added ingredient of having to assertively and openly set sexual limits with their partners may diminish the anxiety-reducing effect of sex. Such a shift may prompt them to resist adopting safe-sex techniques. But, in the long run, not having to worry about infecting someone else or getting infected (or re-infected) will become a decided benefit of practicing safe sex. In addition, with some practice and willingness to experiment, individuals will likely find that safe sex can fulfill many of the needs that their former sexual practices did. Individuals who have continuing problems with adapting to safe sex, or who feel that they are sexually compulsive, may want to seek special help. They may be helped by the techniques used for other compulsive disorders like alcohol and substance abuse, over-eating, etc. Such groups as Sex and Love Anonymous, designed for the sexually compulsive person, may be especially helpful.

Intimacy

Intimate relationships fulfill basic human desires for love and affection. Relationships can also answer sexual needs and be a haven from the fears, anxieties, and general complications of the AIDS crisis. Concern about AIDS has created an atmosphere wherein more emphasis and more peer pressure are exerted on individuals to become part of a couple. For those individuals who have been in few relationships in the past, this new prospect may involve learning a new set of skills, such as cooperative living. More basic for many, however, is learning to deal with fears of intimacy. Those who have had a history of being in intimate relationships but are not presently in one may feel confused and frustrated about finding a new and appropriate partner. Many people in this category previously relied on making social contacts in bars; now they may wish to find new ways to meet people. Many now look to such social groups as hiking clubs, athletic clubs, volunteer work, and even bingo parties, as opportunities to meet a partner.

Another group concerned with intimacy are those who are already in relationships. For some of them, having sex outside the primary relationship was used by one or both partners to alleviate pressure or sexual boredom within the relationship, or to lessen external pressures. Many of these couples, concerned about the risks of AIDS, have now considered closing their open relationship. This sometimes creates difficult expectations: the relationship alone is now expected to meet many needs previously satisfied elsewhere. Sometimes couples will seek what is called "couple counseling," allowing them to talk with a therapist together and focus on improving their relationship.

Emotional Support

Personal and emotional support is often best provided by families, friends, spouses, and lovers. Most importantly, perhaps, is the kind of support that can come from fellow persons with AIDS. Support groups have become an intrinsic part of the treatment of people with AIDS. Knowing that others face similar problems, fear similar fears, and share similar joys is comforting to each of us. This is especially necessary for individuals who are isolated from society as are many people with AIDS. Frequently, those who are newly diagnosed express initial hesitation about joining a support group. This is understandable, since going to one of these groups can be a frightening experience the first time. Attending the group means that one accepts the diagnosis and is willing to be confronted by the words, faces, and physical conditions of the other group members and by whatever the future may bring. Support groups provide an opportunity for those people who have been diagnosed with AIDS to discuss their varied reactions in a safe atmosphere with people who truly understand, at a feeling level, as they share their experience. With time comes trust; friendships form; and people can begin to move to a point of acceptance of their diagnosis and illness.

Physical contact in these support groups is of great importance to people with AIDS, for they may not be getting much physical comfort elsewhere due to people's unjustified and ill-informed fears of casual contagion. Groups can also help people express their anger and resentment as a result of having lost friends, lovers, homes, and being asked to leave bars, restaurants, and even juries. Group discussions may center around any of the following: medical information, decisions and treatment, financial planning, disability applications, discriminatory treatment, and needs for supportive physical contact. Role models for dealing with adversity often emerge.

Support groups can provide a safe and useful mechanism for friends, family, and lovers of people with AIDS to share their experiences as well. While not directly afflicted with AIDS, these individuals may share many of the concerns and fears of the individual who actually has AIDS. Topics discussed might include fear of contagion, fear of death or grieving, reduced or altered social life, health concerns, or obsessional thoughts about AIDS.

AIDS Project Los Angeles Support Groups

David Epstein, Ph.D.

For persons with AIDS, AIDS Project Los Angeles (APLA) provides support groups that are similar to those offered by other AIDS organizations around the country. Within APLA's groups, members are encouraged to live with AIDS by finding and developing new meaning in their lives, to accept support and help as they maintain a sense of mastery over their own lives, and to strive toward self-enhancement.

Often when individuals are confronted with the possibility of their death, the meaning of their lives becomes a focus of attention. Whether people believe that they have forty years or four months to live, we encourage them to find value in living in the present. For one group member, this translates into truly enjoying his friends and family; for another, it means accepting himself and his homosexuality.

Group members are encouraged to discuss their medical treatment and are supported in their efforts to cope with the illness by consulting physicians, psychotherapists, nutritionists, and other health-care professionals. Some members find it helpful to "mentally fight" the illness through visual imagery in addition to working with health-care professionals.

As noted earlier, AIDS can psychologically wear someone down. Group members, therefore, are encouraged to nurture themselves or to do things which will bring joy to their lives. Many group members who have had to deny themselves a great deal, or who have suffered losses in several areas of their lives, report having renewed faith in themselves and their own inner resources. Several members have been able to finally do positive things for themselves which they had put off for years prior to their diagnosis of AIDS. All group members are actively encouraged to support one another in not succumbing to guilt or self-blame. Some group members have found comfort in the book *When Bad Things Happen to Good People* (Kushner, 1981). Family members have found comfort in a more recent book, *When Someone You Love Has AIDS: A Book of Hope for Family and Friends* (Moffatt, 1986).

AIDS is a difficult life situation for all involved—from the individual diagnosed with AIDS to the health-care professional caring for him or her. To conclude, it is understandable that those diagnosed with AIDS—and even those who are not—experience tremendous distress and frustration as a result of the syndrome. It is important to seek and accept support from those who care and share your concerns. There are people who will listen and be physically available to you with whom you can socialize and share, helping you to survive this time of crisis.

[Editor's note: There are a variety of ongoing support groups for persons with AIDS, or those personally affected by AIDS. For details, consult the Resource Directory in Section Ten, APPENDICES.]

Coping with Stress

Jaak Hamilton, M.F.C.C., and Scott Sherman, Ph.D.

[Editor's note: The day-to-day stress of living with AIDS is an important factor in the lives of the AIDS person, his friends, and family. Managing stress, therefore, becomes an important aspect of managing the AIDS illness.]

When considering the issues of stress—its control and reduction, as well as its health impact—it is important to understand that there are varying levels and types of stress. The purpose of this article is to offer some suggestions about how to (1) recognize situations that cause stress; (2) recognize when you are feeling stressed; and then (3) determine positive actions to eliminate or minimize the impact of the stress-inducing situation.

Stress manifests in different ways and in many settings. It can occur because of situations over which we have little or no control. Examples of this might include natural disasters (floods, earthquakes, etc.), traffic problems, or power failures. Such episodes often leave us feeling victimized. *Understanding* and *accepting* that we have little control over these situations is the first step; the second is learning to *cope* with them.

Another form of stress over which we *do* have some control is the stress we often bring upon ourselves. This is where it is helpful to take preventive steps and learn how to control or minimize stressful situations.

One approach to stress management is to know *your* early warning signs of stress. There are many ways to do this, and they may be different for every individual. In fact, levels of stress and what is stressful differ for each person. For some people, stress can be a motivating factor, while for others it may inhibit or limit their ability to function. You must know how stress works for *you* and when it rises beyond a workable level, hit your red flag and set a stress management plan into action.

Signs of stress can manifest physically or psychologically. The following are common:

Physical Signs of Stress

Tension headache
Tight neck or shoulders
Eye strain
Upset in usual sleep pattern
Upset stomach, "butterflies"
Disrupted eating patterns
Rash
Hyperventilation (short, rapid, shallow breaths; panting)

Psychological/Emotional Signs of Stress

Feeling:
— tense or edgy
— depressed or blue
Short-tempered or unusually impatient
Disoriented, scattered
Short concentration span

Stress management takes many forms; you will have to determine which is most appropriate or useful for *you*. Perhaps one of the most effective (and healthful) means of controlling stress is physical exercise. This does not mean a ten-mile jog or an hour of wrestling. Do what you can, what your health allows. A casual stroll can be as beneficial as a light jog; or try swimming (easy on the body), bike riding, a short hike in pleasant surroundings. There are endless alternatives.

Other activities that help relieve your mind are also helpful. Watch television, or sit in a jacuzzi. (In lieu of a jacuzzi, try a hot bubble bath. Don't laugh—it works beautifully. It's cheap and almost everyone has a bath tub.)

Get involved in activities which are fun and enjoyable. How about cards or a game of Trivial Pursuit? Many cities have clubs which offer options like movie-going, bridge, or bowling. Check out your area and interests. If you do not find what you like, take some initiative. Start an activity yourself. Do not wait for someone to take the ball; run with it yourself.

Other methods of stress reduction might include mental or spiritual exercises such as hypnosis or meditation. Biofeedback is an excellent tool. (You can purchase a manual biofeedback machine for $15 at Radio Shack.) Guided imagery and deep muscle relaxation are also very useful. You can learn to do these on your own or purchase tapes to aid you. Deep breathing, a preliminary for most relaxation exercises, is easy and you can do it anytime and anywhere.

As has been seen in gerontology studies, pets can play an enormous role in reducing stress and bringing calm into chaos. Whether it be the stroking of a dog's fur, the playfulness of a cat, the laziness of a fish, pets can be hypnotic and relaxing. *A precautionary note:* Before selecting a pet, immune-suppressed individuals should check with their doctor. Some animals and their care may put people with AIDS or AIDS-related complex at risk of developing certain infections.

Additionally, there are some structured exercises that can help prevent or control stress. You might list activities or individuals you find particularly stressful, or make a list of activities on a timeline so that you can put events in perspective. Then see how you can restructure these activities to make them more workable. Plan ahead so that you can take pressure off, and pace yourself.

Above all, cultivate those people in your life who are supportive and healthy. Have more dinners with friends. Have people over to play Monopoly, cards, or just a night of television.

It is imperative that we all understand that stress can undermine our health—spiritually, emotionally, mentally, and physically; we must guard against it. We must treat ourselves kindly, with care and love. We must attend to and address our needs on all levels. We are holistic entities and must not ignore one facet of our lives while taking care of another.

Surround yourself with positive influences and thoughts. Make your activities work *for* you, not against you. Find time to be alone, peaceful, and learn to enjoy that which is you.

From the Heart: The Family's Response

Michael Helquist

If someone in your family has contracted AIDS or ARC or has been exposed to the AIDS virus, you may feel that your life suddenly resembles a roller-coaster ride. Not only will you have a great number of questions related to medicine and illness, but you will most likely feel intense fear, anger, and sadness, as well as confusion and frustration. It is a very difficult experience to care for someone who has a life-threatening illness like AIDS.

Your first concern will probably focus on the condition, both physical and emotional, of your loved one. People with AIDS usually experience overwhelming personal changes when they are diagnosed with this life-threatening illness. Often their lives change radically. Health, social life, and expectations for the future are altered. Some must also adjust to the loss of their jobs, their independence, their homes; to reduced finances, to lengthy hospital stays, and to tiring treatment progress. Not understanding what is happening to their bodies now and not knowing what will happen next may cause severe emotional

---

This article is based on a booklet, *The Family Guide to AIDS*, published by the San Francisco AIDS Foundation.

strain. Additionally, they must confront feelings of isolation from friends, loss of independence, and fear of dying. Spouses, parents, brothers and sisters, other relatives, lovers and friends become perhaps more important than ever before for someone with AIDS.

The Family of the Person with AIDS

Many people have developed an "extended family" comprised of a number of close relationships with other men and women friends. This network of relationships frequently becomes a valuable source of support, especially during difficult times. You may find these close friends to be a source of comfort and help for yourself as well. One mother who traveled from her home on the East Coast to San Francisco to visit her son with AIDS found the presence of his friends very reassuring. In her words:

> Once we were at the hospital, I saw all these friends come by to see him. I realized that he also has family here in San Francisco. He calls his friends his family, and I understand that now. I felt all the love coming to him. And I felt reassured. I knew he was in good hands.

When you need to talk with someone who knows your loved one well, these may be the people to whom you can turn. They may be very willing to assist with completing insurance forms, household chores, and bedside care. If you're unfamiliar with the city you're visiting and need assistance with transportation, or need help in getting answers about available services, these individuals may be a ready resource. If they are unable to provide the help you need, the community agencies listed in the appendix of this guide are a good resource.

You Can Help

Health professionals who work specifically with those who have life-threatening illnesses suggest that the single most important thing a family can offer is a willingness to go through this experience with their loved one. Yet your willingness to stay nearby through this difficult time may cause you a great amount of distress and worry. Your own health and well-being continue to be very important. You may want to speak with someone who can be supportive of you. It may help to acknowledge your worries and fears with your loved one as part of going through the experience together. You may also want to confide in someone else. Many people have a tendency to ignore their own feelings while they focus on the person who is ill. While some of your own needs may be set aside temporarily, remember how important your good health is not only to the person who is ill, but also to your family and friends.

Individuals with AIDS don't want to think and talk about the disease all the time. It is often important for them to feel a part of everyday events, and to hear the daily news of family and friends. Remember, too, that a sense of humor can be invaluable for keeping some perspective about an AIDS diagnosis. Someone with a life-threatening disease can feel isolated and suddenly cut off from a life that preceded the disease.

The most important time becomes the present moment. Encourage your loved one to do all that can be done each day. Do not underestimate the effects of the illness, but avoid being overly protective. Encourage active involvement in the family's discussions and activities. If you're visiting in the hospital, or even at home, realize that there will be natural lulls in the conversation. You do not have to say anything. Relax with the silence. Your presence will often be more important than your words. Touching and smiling can convey much affection and reassurance. Your loved one will want to know that this illness has not altered your feelings of love and affection.

Almost every person diagnosed with AIDS is determined to recover and regain good health. Many see themselves as fighting for their lives, taking an active role in getting well again. Most want and need the support of their families in this effort. Many people with AIDS come to recognize that they have a life-threatening illness while they reject the notion that they are dying of AIDS.

One person with AIDS has written: "I don't feel like a patient—passive, fearful, and immobilized. Rather, I am an active participant in the fight for my health, working with the doctors, molding my recovery, acknowledging my fears, and communicating as best I can."

You can help support recovery with a focus on getting well rather than on remaining ill.

Ways of Coping

The diagnosis of a life-threatening illness comes as a shock. It is not unusual for the person with the illness to feel intense anger, fear, confusion, and a general sense of loss.

These feelings may at times come out unexpectedly and forcibly. Since there is often an expectation that feelings of love within the family will remain constant no matter what, you and other family members may be the only persons considered a safe "target" for angry outbursts. An AIDS diagnosis may at times be too much to handle for the person with the disease. They may desire to be taken care of and to give in to a sense of helplessness. Family members are frequently challenged to provide support without being over-protective. Remember, the person with AIDS cannot be rescued from the disease. You can offer support and a shoulder to lean on, and perhaps to cry on, but the individual will need to develop a personal method of coping with the diagnosis.

Although AIDS has been contracted by some heterosexual men and women, the majority of people in the United States with AIDS are gay and bisexual men at this time. This does not mean that AIDS is a "gay disease." However, for some parents it does prompt discussions about their son's homosexuality. For a great variety of reasons, many men may have not previously revealed their homosexuality to their parents. To undertake such discussions now, while coping with the diagnosis of a serious disease, can be very difficult. As a parent you may feel shocked, embarrassed, hurt, and angry. You may not know what to tell friends and neighbors. You will perhaps want to confide in a trusted friend or perhaps in a pastor, minister, or rabbi. You may also feel proud of your son's decision to live his life in a manner that is true to his own feelings. For many parents what becomes most important at this time is the love they share with their son. With those feelings expressed and confirmed, other concerns can fall into some perspective.

There are organizations to contact to discuss your concerns as parents and family members; these include Mothers of AIDS Patients (see the Resource Directory in the Appendices of this guide), and local chapters of Parents and Friends of Lesbians and Gays (PFLAG), as well as Parents and Friends of Gays.

As more heterosexual individuals develop AIDS symptoms, family members should not assume that the individual has a certain lifestyle (homosexuality or needle-sharing drug use). Instead they should be open to their loved one's explanation of his or her possible exposure and invite sensitive discussion of how that person is adapting to the diagnosis.

Some people diagnosed with AIDS develop more serious medical consequences than others. When tests, treatments, and hospitalizations become frequent, the life of the person with AIDS and the lives of loved ones lose their normal daily patterns and often become very difficult. If you find yourself in these situations, the following ideas may be helpful.

Patient Advocacy. Confronting the medical establishment of hospitals, clinics, and doctors' offices can be overwhelming for a person in good health. The unknowns about AIDS often mean that there are many tests, reports, and opinions. It can be helpful to have one or two others who are close to your loved one to listen to the doctor's reports, ask questions, and take notes.

Information can help reduce the fear of the unknown. You can also help establish a rapport with the medical staff in the clinic, doctor's office, or hospital. Let the staff know you are interested, and that you will politely, but firmly, follow through to meet the needs of the patient. Become a partner in the medical care, and ask questions when you need to. There is reason to be assertive in the hospital. All institutions have their own daily routines that seem to work best for that facility. Sometimes the routine may not be the best for the patient. For example, a patient's room does not have to be cleaned at a given moment; the staff can be asked to wait another twenty minutes. Your loved one can ask for maximum privacy, not only from visitors, but also from staff.

The Hospital Room. In the hospital room, you may want to make the surroundings as pleasant as possible. Flowers, music, balloons, food you have prepared, and whatever else might be pleasing to your loved one—all are appropriate. Sometimes it may be more comforting to the patient to have silence in the room, and some visitors may have to learn to relax with this request. Quiet background music, perhaps a light massage, or just quietly holding hands can be very soothing for the patient. If the room is being shared with another patient, be considerate of that person's needs as well. If your loved one is in the hospital for an extended stay, be sure to let others, friends and relatives, assist you with the visiting. Take a break from your visits; perhaps get some fresh air by going for a walk. You need your moments of relief and rest.

Getting Out Information. It might help for one or two friends to serve as a contact for the larger group of friends and acquaintances who are concerned about medical developments. These contacts may want to make their phone numbers available for others to call them. There's a delicate balance between getting overwhelmed with questions and disseminating needed information. Some families find it helpful to have a telephone answering machine with a message that is updated on a regular basis.

Insurance Forms, etc. It may not be possible or desirable for the person with AIDS to be responsible for completing all the insurance forms, disability forms, et cetera. One other person could relieve much pressure by assuming this role of "taking care of business." Perhaps someone could "monitor" non-medical mail for important bills, checks, and letters.

Medical Issues. You or someone else could keep track of the medications; which drugs are to be taken and when. Questions may arise: Is it all right to take another pain killer now? When was the last one taken? You should also know whom to call in time of emergency.

Personal Affairs. Getting personal affairs in order is a good idea for even the most healthy among us. Does your loved one have a current will? Do you know where it is kept? Is there a list of bank accounts, charge accounts, outstanding loans, etc? Have you considered obtaining a durable power of attorney status which allows someone else to make medical decisions for you if you are unable to do so for yourself? If you have an extended stay in the hospital, have you arranged for someone to take care of your bills and other such matters? (See Section Seven, A PRACTICAL PERSPECTIVE.)

Emotional Stress. The strain of serious illness can be intense for everyone involved. Much of this experience can be shared with a spouse, other family members, or close friends. But a lot of it may be too personal to share. This can be very frustrating. You may find that these difficult events cause a great deal of strain for you with your other relationships. While some families have found that these difficulties eventually forge stronger bonds of communication and love, your own stress may prompt great anxiety for both you and your loved ones. You may feel insistent that your loved one eat more or sleep more—*anything* to get better. Your feelings are natural, but you have to take care of yourself as well. An awareness of these natural responses and a willingness to communicate may prove helpful. A sense of humor may also help you get through these stressful times. Sometimes remembering to take a deep breath and to step back from the immediacy of the situation allows for some beneficial perspective.

Do not be afraid to seek professional help to cope with stress for yourself, the loved one with AIDS, and family members. Often hospitals have social workers or therapists on staff. Some community-based AIDS service organizations also provide such services.

Fear of AIDS. Any new disease that is life-threatening, with no known cure, can be frightening. The media's frequent reports about AIDS often stir up unwarranted fears among the public. Medical experts agree that AIDS is not easily transferred to another person. There is no reason to fear you are "catching AIDS" by being in the same room with someone who has AIDS, or by using the same linens or kitchen utensils after proper washing. *There is no reason to believe that AIDS is spread by casual household contact.* Others—relatives, neighbors, friends—may need more information about AIDS and to correct misinformation. It's important that visitors observe guidelines for infection control (see the "Home Care" and "Hygiene" segments of Section Six). The person with AIDS does not need to have to combat even the common viruses and infections, like colds, coughs, and the flu, while trying to improve an impaired immune system. Advise visitors to postpone their visit or visit by telephone if they are not feeling well themselves.

You may not fear "catching AIDS" yourself, but may be frightened by the outcome this illness may bring for your loved one. The uncertainty is very stressful; you may fear losing your loved one. It's important to recognize your fears and talk about them when possible. Your support is needed; fear can sometimes block expressions of understanding and affection. These are gifts you can offer to your special person.

Youth at Risk

Marcia Quackenbush, M.S., M.F.C.C.

The risks to adolescents of coming into contact with the AIDS virus are the same as for adults; thus, the sexual and drug use practices of teenagers provide a clear avenue for the transmission of AIDS. Prevention efforts, however, are complicated by particular developmental issues that occur for adolescents. Nevertheless, young people need and deserve AIDS prevention education that is carefully planned and consistently implemented.

Scope of Risk

At present, very few adolescents have actually been diagnosed with AIDS. The Centers for Disease Control (CDC) report less than 1 percent of total cases are among 13–19 year olds. However, the main routes of infection—unsafe sexual contact and needle-sharing drug use—involve activities practiced by a high proportion of teenagers. For example, 50 percent of teenage women in high school have had sexual intercourse, and 16 percent (more than 1.5 million) report having had four or more partners. In addition, there are 1.2 million teenage pregnancies in the United States annually (about 3,000 conceptions

This article first appeared in *FOCUS: A Review of AIDS Research*, February 1987, Volume 2, Number 3.

per day),[1] and health officials estimate that one in seven teenagers currently has a sexually transmitted disease (STD).[2] The same activities that cause pregnancies and most STDs can also expose an individual to AIDS.

While there are no national statistics on IV-drug use among teenagers, conservative estimates suggest more than 200,000 high school students have used heroin. Millions more have used cocaine, stimulants, or other opiates,[3] all substances that can be used intravenously. Furthermore, youths who have dropped out of high school may have higher rates of IV-drug use than those in school, and 25 percent of all students will drop out before high school graduation.

Finally, due to the long incubation period for AIDS, averaging over six years at present,* many individuals diagnosed in their twenties (about 21 percent of total cases reported, some cases as of January 1987), were probably infected during their teens.

Developmental Issues

Popular attitudes, as well as some traditional teachings, suggest that adolescence is a time of turmoil, disequilibrium, and distress. In fact, many more recent theorists have discarded this idea. In an impressive twenty-year retrospective study, Offer, Ostrov, and Howard[4] provide data showing that most adolescents feel strong, happy, and self-confident, and they remark that "the turmoil theory is simply wrong in that it is not applicable to the vast majority of adolescents."

This absence of turmoil for most adolescents does not necessarily mean there is an absence of danger, and the issues of normal adolescent development present special challenges to the teen counselor or educator attempting to provide AIDS prevention information. Such work is certainly more arduous with the disturbed or chaotic adolescent client. Some of these developmental issues and the manner in which they might have an impact on AIDS education efforts are discussed below.

Cognitive and Emotional Development. Adolescence is a time of increased focus on personal identity and strong identification with the peer group. More sophisticated mental capabilities develop, allowing young people to begin to see their parents as separate individuals and to see errors in their reasoning.

---

* Editor's note: Current research indicates that the incubation period may be as long as ten years.

Teenagers experiment with greater independence, and many begin, for the first time, to identify moral codes differing from those of their parents. This usually healthy questioning (and sometimes distrust) of parents and other adults allows the young person to refine further a sense of self. Unfortunately, it can also lead to frustration for the educator hoping to persuade the teen of the risks of AIDS (or of smoking, drinking, and other activities which threaten well-being).

Youths generally use two important frameworks to view themselves in the world. One is a somewhat egocentric, present-time orientation—it is difficult for the young person to imagine a future very distant from today. The other framework is a sense of personal invulnerability. Teenagers often think, I can take risks and nothing bad will happen to me. These attitudes present obstacles for education about risks for a lethal disease with a six-year, possibly even ten-year, incubation period.

For the youth with emotional, psychological, social, or family problems, all these factors may become exaggerated and sometimes harmful. This young person may feel able to establish a sense of separateness from parents and other adults only through acting out behavior such as dangerous use of drugs or alcohol, sexual promiscuity, or delinquency. The sense of personal invulnerability may lead to extreme risk-taking behavior, and the present-time orientation may be transformed into a nihilistic, self-destructive posture. Those working in mental health setting, detention facilities, school counseling, or public health clinics are likely to see many such adolescents.

Experimentation is a typical behavior of adolescents. Normal development often includes experimentation with drugs, sex, styles of dress, ways of talking, and different friendships. These activities serve the individual in the search for self-identity. For the troubled adolescent, experiments may become habits, and the fluid search for self may become rigid and destructive.

The cautions of AIDS education must be integrated into this practice of normal experimentation, and educators must expect that both normal and troubled teens will continue experimental behavior of one sort or another. Healthy options for experimentation will be more helpful than unreasonable and unrealistic prohibitions against personal exploration.

Social, Behavioral, and Physiological Development. Increased identity with the peer group may lead to changes in teen activities. Parents' opinions about some issues become less important than those of friends. Interest develops in the opposite sex, both as "dates" and as friends. Childhood pastimes are often abandoned in favor of talking, "hanging out," and establishing group cohesion through shared activities. While much of the social development of adolescents is self-centered, there may also be increased interest in world events and greater concern for community welfare.

Peer attitudes regarding sexual activity and drug use have a powerful influence on personal decisions about engaging in these forms of behavior. It is difficult to feel one is the only individual in the crowd doing or not doing something. The AIDS educator who makes recommendations that go against the ethic of the teen's peer community may find it difficult to be persuasive.

Adolescents discover that parents are not omniscient; thus they can choose to withhold knowledge from parents, and activities can be carried out in secret. Furthermore, the parent usually cannot physically restrain the adolescent child. The possibility then arises of pursuing independent behavior or those disapproved of by parents and other adults. This can include sexual and drug-use activities.

The sexual maturation of teens, combined with their cognitive and emotional development, usually creates greater interest in sexual issues. It certainly contributes to the possibility of sexual activity taking place. For this reason alone it is essential to educate youth about AIDS and to encourage teens who are sexual to adhere to safe-sex guidelines.

Family Relationships

The teen years are times when unresolved issues between children and parents, especially regarding power and control, are likely to arise again. Parents of adolescents sometimes have their own mid-life concerns with issues about health, professional success, and sexual attractiveness. They may project resentments, vicarious desires, or unrealistic expectations onto children just beginning their adult lives. In such families, teens may act out, usually in the areas of sexual activity or alcohol and drug use. Therapeutic or educational interventions may help divert such behavior patterns or channel them into non-risk choices.

AIDS Education

Runaways, Street Youth, and Incarcerated Juveniles. Estimates of the number of runaway minors in the United States annually range from 500,000 to 1.25 million. Many join the ranks of street youth, surviving by whatever means possible, including prostitution and drug dealing. Rates of sexual activity, drug use, STDs, suicide attempts, and encounters with the legal system are higher for runaways than for youth from intact homes. These young people are often actually "throwaways," discarded from chaotic, abusive families. Prostitution (often involving unsafe sex) is linked with survival, and IV-drug use is frequently practiced by peers. These youth often fully expect to have limited lifespans; their AIDS-related risks are high; and AIDS prevention messages are easily lost or disregarded in the drama of more immediate crises—where to sleep that night, how to obtain food for the day, or when the next fix will arrive.

Youth service workers who have regular contact with street youth are the most effective bearers of AIDS education. They have found that when educational efforts are consistent and persistent, certain ethics about risk activities can be changed among those in the street community. Peer influence is immensely important on the street, and the communication network is extensive; for each individual reached directly, five or ten others may hear the message. Such youth service workers need specific training about outlining methods and content for AIDS prevention with street youth, sharing information updates, and providing other requested consultations.

Youth detained by juvenile authorities are a captive audience, providing many opportunities for education. These individuals usually respond well to personal attention at medical clinics, and they are receptive to expressions of interest in their well-being. The boredom experienced by juvenile detainees works in favor of the educator, since they may enjoy almost any distraction, even if it means talking to someone about AIDS risks.

AIDS information for street youth and incarcerated juveniles must be accurate, simple, explicit, and direct. Verbal education is preferable to written materials. Many of these youth are learning-disabled or have other problems with reading. Language and cultural differences must be considered with programs developed specifically for communities with a primary language other than English.

Health Clinic Visits and Private Physician Patients. Young people seeking health consultation or treatment from family physicians or through private or public clinics can also receive AIDS prevention education, regardless of presenting concerns. Written materials (brochures and posters) could be available in waiting rooms. Discreet wallet-sized cards printed with resource information numbers and safe-sex guidelines can be distributed during office visits. As a natural part of a general health assessment, a sexual history can be obtained.

AIDS information is important even for teens who currently are not sexually active; at some future time they almost certainly will be. Again, materials and verbal presentations must be simple and explicit. Similar guidelines can be used at mental health clinics as well as drug and alcohol treatment centers.

Public and Private School Students. Schools have the opportunity to provide integrated educational programs spanning the child's school career. In early grades, the nature of communicable disease can be discussed along with family life education focusing on friendships, family relationships, and the basics of reproduction. Pre-adolescents (fifth and sixth graders) are ready for more sophisticated information about intimacy, sexuality, and disease prevention. At this age, children are quite receptive to information about sexuality, perhaps more so than in adolescence, when their own emerging sexual feelings may lead to greater resistance in sex education classes. Starting this education early lays the foundation for continued mention of AIDS prevention throughout middle and high school, and it provides needed information to those who may drop out long before graduation.

By middle school age, a significant number of students are nearing or, have already begun, sexually active lives. AIDS education must be provided at this level if prevention efforts are to be effective. The lessons should be specific, direct, and explicit about means of transmission as well as methods of prevention. Education for high school students can continue along this line, with more sophisticated materials appropriate for the more mature student.

AIDS can be taught to middle and high school students in a variety of creative and effective manners. AIDS-specific teaching units appropriate for many different classes, such as family life, history, social studies, psychology, or science, can help teenagers by offering the basics about AIDS prevention several times and in different settings over the course of their schooling. Current research suggests that exposure to health curricula in schools does affect students' attitudes, knowledge, and behavior,[5] and early surveys of students' knowledge about AIDS reveal better understanding among those who have had classes on AIDS prevention.[6]

Parent participation in the development of AIDS education plans for the schools should also be considered, both to review materials and to provide support for programs.

Conclusion

Clearly, teenagers engage in activities that may put them at risk for AIDS. Education about AIDS prevention may be difficult with some youths because of their surfacing independence, rebellion, distrust of adults, present-time orientation, and myths of personal invulnerability. It is essential to acknowledge that the AIDS-risk activities of teenagers are not the special province of "bad kids," troubled youth, or the emotionally disturbed. AIDS prevention education must become a standard part of service contact with all youth, and this knowledge must become a common and natural element of all that young people know.

Footnote References

1. *Teenage Pregnancy: The Problem That Hasn't Gone Away*; New York, Alan Guttmacher Institute, 1981.

2. Lumiere R., Cook S. *Healthy Sex*; New York, Simon & Schuster, 1983.

3. Johnston L.D., O'Mally P.M., Bachman J.G. *Use of Licit and Illicit Drugs by America's High School Students 1975–1984*; U.S. Department of Health and Human Services, 1985; DHHS Publications No. (ADM) 85-1394.

4. Offer D., Ostrov E., Howard K. *The Adolescent: A Psychological Self-Portrait*; New York, Basic Books, 1981.

5. "The Effectiveness of School Health Education." MMWR, 35 (38), September 26, 1986. p. 593-595.

6. DiClemente R.J., Zorn J., and Temoshok L. "Adolescents and AIDS: A Survey of Knowledge, Attitudes, and Beliefs About AIDS in San Francisco." AJPH, 1986, 76, 12.

AIDS in Children: Social, Psychological, and Ethical Aspects

Graeme Hanson, M.D.

The virus that causes AIDS has made its devastation known in the child and adolescent population, although in relatively low numbers to date. Children and teenagers are at risk for infection with the AIDS virus from three different sources: maternal transmission, blood transfusions and use of blood products, sexual activity, and shared needles during IV-drug use. Very young children may have been exposed in utero or in the perinatal period (that time before, during, and immediately after birth) or as a result of transfusions. The school-age child may have been infected through transfusions of blood or blood products (for example, the child with hemophilia), and the teenager may have been exposed through sexual activity or through sharing needles during IV-drug use.

This article first appeared in *FOCUS: A Review of AIDS Research*, Volume 1, Number 5, April 1986.

The increasing appearance of AIDS, AIDS-related complex (ARC), or the AIDS antibody in children confronts us with profound and difficult ethical issues. In addition, the potential is great for serious and long-lasting psychological consequences for the child, the family, and for society as a whole.

As the impact of AIDS on children becomes more apparent, at least three crucial needs can and often will conflict with each other: (1) the need for research to provide the knowledge and understanding of this disease in order to find an adequate treatment and cure; (2) the need for humane and sensitive treatment as well as protection for the individual child; and (3) the need to protect other people and to prevent the spread of the disease. When these needs conflict, there are no ready solutions. Nevertheless, in this emotionally charged crisis we must be able to question and consider the results of our actions and the motivating factors behind them.

It is important to understand the powerful emotional responses that AIDS evokes in adults. These reactions result from the associations of AIDS with sexuality, homosexuality, illicit drug use, promiscuity, and prostitution. Each of these elicits strong societal condemnation, prejudice, and discrimination. The power of fear and prejudice cannot be underestimated when we attempt to find a rational approach to this tragic condition. These feelings can affect not only the general public but also care-givers, service providers, public officials, and scientists.

"AIDS hysteria" results from a complex combination of the usual fear of the mysterious and unknown and the very real consequences of AIDS. One aspect of fear and prejudice in these circumstances is the psychological need to segregate out of fear of contamination. In the AIDS context, this psychological need becomes intricately interwoven with real threats of contagion and the uncertainties about the spread of the disease.

These aspects of the emotional reactions of adults are important for several reasons: (1) The social and psychological implications for children who have AIDS, ARC, or who are seropositive, meaning that they have tested positive on the AIDS antibody test, will depend to a large extent on the reactions and responses of the adults in the child's life; (2) policies, regulations, and procedures that profoundly affect the lives of children are promulgated by adults who are subject to these psychological influences; and (3) fear and prejudice are difficult to counter with reason.

Efforts to educate the public are critically important; they must be more intensive than might be needed in a medical crisis without such complex psychological and social overtones. The implications of the social, psychological, and ethical factors of AIDS may differ somewhat among children with AIDS, children with ARC, and those who are seropositive. The major issues, however, are similar for each group.

Questions of Confidentiality

Due to the intense emotional climate surrounding the AIDS epidemic, one of the most important issues for the child with AIDS, ARC, or confirmed exposure is the matter of confidentiality. Questions immediately arise: Who needs to know? Who needs to know what? And for what purpose? These are questions that must be faced. Does the potential good of revealing this information outweigh the potential harm and how can the confidentiality be ensured? Who controls this information?

Opinions vary greatly on these matters; different jurisdictions are already enacting very different kinds of regulations for reporting, dissemination of information, and quarantine options. (A public opinion poll conducted last December by the Los Angeles Times regarding AIDS in adults found that 48 percent favored mandatory identification cards for people with positive results to the AIDS antibody test. Fifty-one percent supported quarantine; 15 percent supported tatooing people with AIDS. Interestingly, 55 percent said they would send their child to a classroom even if a classmate had AIDS.)

Vaccines and Foster Homes

For the infant and very young child infected with the virus, there are certain important precautions necessary for the protection of the child. The young child with a compromised immune system probably should not be immunized with live virus as is found in mumps, measles, and some polio immunizations. Therefore, the caretakers of an AIDS antibody positive child need to do all they can to protect the child from exposure to infection, especially to certain childhood diseases like chickenpox, mumps, and measles. The primary caretaker and the physician of the child need to know if the child has been infected. The situation becomes complicated if one considers that many of the affected babies are born to drug-addicted mothers and are likely to be placed in foster care. Therefore, the foster parents will need to know. In those cases, how many foster parents will want to care for such children? What impact will this have on the foster-care system already significantly lacking in adequate foster homes?

If the child develops AIDS while in foster care, the likelihood of that child being returned to the system is great, creating yet another trauma for an already vulnerable and compromised child.

Social and Psychological Implications

For the seropositive young child living with his or her natural parents, the parents will live with a painful uncertainty, a kind of medical and psychological time bomb. How will this affect the parents' relationship with their child? If the child develops AIDS, the parents, especially the mother, may be overwhelmed by a sense of guilt for having infected the child.

For the school-age child, the social implications of having AIDS, ARC, or seropositivity are of special significance. This is an age when being able to attend school, to participate in activities with other children, to be acceptable and included in a group are very important. If children are excluded from school or from certain activities, they will likely experience serious psychological and social adjustment difficulties.

Medical experts generally recommend that children with AIDS be allowed to attend school. If the condition of these children becomes known to their classmates, they will likely be subject to teasing and discrimination. And if these affected children are excluded from school or from other activities, they will most likely be encouraged to keep confidential the reason for their exclusion. Having to keep this kind of secret can have detrimental results in the development of a positive sense of self, of being acceptable, and of being integrated. These children and their parents will need help in adjusting to this situation. Parents will especially need advice and counseling regarding how they can discuss this complex matter with their child.

Teenagers are at risk for AIDS through sexual activity and through sharing needles during IV-drug use. The question of screening at-risk teens is a difficult one. If the information obtained by such a screening would be clinically useful, then screening might be advisable. At present the disadvantages appear to outweigh the advantages. This is especially true for those teens who are probably the most at risk—the homeless runaways who are vulnerable to drug use and prostitution.

Many of the issues that apply to school-age children also apply to teenagers, such as the problem of being excluded, of being handicapped, and of being socially isolated. In addition, many of the social and psychological factors that affect adults also affect teenagers. If a teen is seropositive and the family is informed, educated guesses about the teen's sexual life or drug use could result in additional psychological trauma for both the teenager and the family.

Teenagers are becoming more aware of and frightened by AIDS. Recently a sixteen-year-old boy became panic stricken after kissing a new girlfriend. He had had some homosexual experiences in the past few months, and suddenly he began to worry that he might be infected and might have infected his girlfriend.

Homeless and runaway youth are especially vulnerable to exposure. They particularly need education and supportive counseling regarding sexual practices and drug use. At the same time, because of their lifestyle, they may be extremely difficult to reach. Explaining the meaning of a positive AIDS antibody test to a teenager could be a very complicated undertaking. The ambiguity and uncertainty may be more than the teen can tolerate. Under such circumstances teenagers tend to act out; the possibility of behavior disturbance, flight into promiscuity, and suicidal activity is great.

Another aspect of AIDS in teens is the unfortunate and painful discrimination that a teen with AIDS may experience from peers. Teenagers frequently struggle with their sexual identity, and prejudice against homosexuality can be profound in this age group. A teenager who has AIDS, ARC, or is seropositive may be seen as tainted or somehow associated with homosexuality in the other healthy teenagers' minds, and consequently face discrimination.

Recommendations

At this point a few recommendations are pertinent. We will need to keep the social and psychological implications clearly in mind when developing public policies. The discussion of school admissions must occur with knowledge of the possible psychological effects on children. Infants of mothers at risk for AIDS may need to be tested for presence of the AIDS antibody to protect those who test seropositive from being immunized with live virus. We will need to provide skilled and trained counselors to help both the children and their families to understand and adjust. All people in a position of caring for children will need education and support, especially teenagers, foster parents, and child-care workers. Parents whose children are in contact with children with AIDS will need information and advice. Most importantly, children themselves will need information and education. Accurate information and understanding are our best tools at this point to help lessen the psychological and social trauma for children with AIDS, ARC, or exposure to the AIDS virus.

When a Friend Has AIDS

While serious illness is a fact of everyday life, AIDS has posed new challenges for everyone involved: not only individuals with AIDS but also their friends. People who are in the prime of their lives have become ill, and their prospects for a long life are severely affected. Their situation is not an isolated one, but is shared by people close to them. When someone you know becomes ill, especially with a serious illness like AIDS, you may feel helpless or inadequate. If this person is a good friend, you may say, "Just call if you need anything." Then out of fear or insecurity, you may dread the call if it comes. Here are some thoughts and suggestions to help you help someone who is ill.

Try not to avoid your friend. Be there—it instills hope. Be the friend, the loved one you've always been, especially now when it is most important.

Touch your friend. A simple squeeze of the hand or a hug can let him or her know that you care. (You needn't be afraid...you cannot contract AIDS by simply touching...and hugs are very reassuring.)

Call and ask if it is okay to come for a visit. Let your friend make the decision. If he or she may not feel up to visitors that day, you can always visit on another occasion. Now is a time when your friendship can help keep loneliness and fear at a distance.

This text was originally printed in a brochure written and developed by Chelsea Psychotherapy Associates of New York City.

Respond to your friend's emotions. Weep with your friend when he or she weeps. Laugh when your friend laughs. It's healthy to share these intimate experiences. They enrich you both.

Call and say you would like to bring a favorite dish. Ask what day and time would be best for you to come. Spend time sharing a meal.

Go for a walk or outing together but ask about and know your friend's limitations.

Offer to help answer any correspondence which may be giving some difficulty or which your friend is avoiding.

Call your friend and find out if anything is needed from the store. Ask for a shopping list and make a delivery to your friend's house.

Celebrate holidays and life with your friend by offering to decorate the home or hospital room. Bring flowers or other special treasures. Include your friend in your holiday festivities. A holiday doesn't have to be marked on a calendar; you can make every day a holiday.

Check in with your friend's spouse, lover, care-partner, roommate, or family member. They may need a break from time to time. Offer to care for the person with AIDS in order to give the loved ones some free time. Invite them out. Remember, they may need someone to talk with as well.

Your friend may be a parent. Ask about the children. Offer to bring them to visit.

Be creative. Bring books, periodicals, taped music, a poster for the wall, home-baked cookies or delicacies to share. All of these can bring warmth and joy.

It's okay to ask about the illness, but be sensitive to whether your friend wants to discuss it. You can find out by asking, "Would you like to talk about how you're feeling?" However, don't pressure.

Like everyone else, a person with AIDS can have both good and bad days. On good days treat your friend as you would any other friend. On the bad days, however, treat your friend with extra care and compassion.

You don't always have to talk. It's okay to sit together silently reading, listening to music, watching television, holding hands. Much can be expressed without words.

Can you take your friend somewhere? Transportation may be needed to a treatment, to the store or bank, to the physician, or perhaps to a movie. How about just a ride to the beach or the park?

Tell your friend how good he or she looks, but only if it is realistic. If your friend's appearance has changed, don't ignore it. Be gentle; yet remember, never lie.

Encourage your friend to make decisions. Illness can cause a loss of control over many aspects of life. Don't deny your friend a chance to make decisions, no matter how simple or silly they may seem to you.

Tell your friend what you'd like to do to help. If your friend agrees to your request, do it. Keep any promises you make.

Be prepared for your friend to get angry with you for no obvious reason, although you feel that you've been there and done everything you could. Remember, anger and frustration are often taken out on the people most loved because it's safe and will be understood.

Gossip can be healthy. Keep your friend up to date on mutual friends and other common interests. Your friend may be tired of talking about symptoms, doctors, and treatments.

What's in the news? Discuss current events. Help keep your friend from feeling that the world is passing by.

Offer to do household chores, perhaps taking out the laundry, washing dishes, watering plants, feeding and walking pets. This may be appreciated more than you realize. However, don't do what your friend wants and can do for him or herself. Ask before doing anything.

Send a card that says, simply, "I care!"

If your friend is religious, ask if you could pray together. Spirituality can be very important at this time.

Don't lecture or direct your anger at your friend if he or she seems to be handling the illness in a way that you think is inappropriate. You may not understand what the feelings are and why certain choices are being made.

Help your friend understand any feeling of blame regarding the illness. Remind your friend that lifestyles don't cause disease, germs do. This may be especially hard for both your friend and you. Help however you can.

If you and your friend are going to engage in sex, be informed about the precautions which make sex safer for both of you. (See "Safe-Sex Guidelines" in Section Five.) Follow them. Be imaginative; touching, stroking, and massage can also be fun.

A loving family member can be a source of strength. Remember that by being a friend or lover you are also a part of the family.

Do not confuse acceptance of the illness with defeat. This acceptance may free your friend and give your friend a sense of his or her own power.

Don't allow your friend or care-partner to become isolated. Let them know about the support groups and other concrete, practical services offered without charge by local AIDS service agencies.

Talk with your friend about the future: tomorrow, next week, next year. It's good to look toward the future without denying the reality of today.

Bring a positive attitude. It's catching.

Finally, take care of yourself! Recognize your own emotions and honor them. Share your grief, anger, feelings of helplessness, or whatever is coming up for you, with others or a support group. Getting the support you need during this crisis will help you to be the real friend for your friend.

People with Hemophilia: Psychosocial Factors

Roslyn Sussman, L.C.S.W.

To better understand the emotional impact of AIDS on the hemophilia community, it is helpful to first look at the psychosocial components of hemophilia itself.

The Diagnosis

The diagnosis of hemophilia, usually confirmed in the child's first year of life, always creates stresses for the family. As the child progresses into adulthood, these stresses may be exacerbated by a number of factors inherent in the illness: pain, bleeding, need for treatment, restricted activity, interruption of school and work, chronic disability, stigmatization and social isolation—all take their toll. These factors strongly influence the self-image and ability of the person with hemophilia and his family to engage in the tasks of everyday living. Occasionally, the patient, the family, or both, may refuse to accept the diagnosis of hemophilia, subsequently neglecting treatment or engaging in rebellious or risk-taking behavior. Other psychological manifestations which may occur are a delay in masculine identification often causing interpersonal problems and a fear of entering into intimate relationships.

Family members manifest their own individual responses to living with hemophilia:

1) Mothers may overprotect or place undue restrictions on the child's activities and decision-making opportunities because of their fears of possible injury or death.

2) Fathers can feel alienated or rejected, and many experience anger as they perceive their sons being overly dependent on their mothers.

3) Siblings often feel frustrated, deprived, or very resentful of the extra attention and apparent favoritism they believe is being accorded the child with hemophilia.

Developing the ability to answer the challenges presented by hemophilia depends on several elements. Each individual's and family's unique combination of useful psychological defenses, coping mechanisms, and knowledge are of primary importance. Also essential for sustaining emotional well-being is the availability of quality medical care, as well as access to educational, vocational, and psychosocial support services.

Many physicians and treatment centers have worked with the hemophilia community for years, watching infants grow into adolescence, boys into adulthood, and men into their time of retirement. They have been instrumental in helping this community of people cope exceedingly well with difficult situations, seeing them achieve in their personal lives equally to any other group in the wider community. Physicians and care-givers have celebrated with their patients when advances in blood products, surgical techniques, and home treatment procedures were achieved, finally enabling persons with hemophilia to anticipate a normal life span.

With all of these breakthroughs it was not surprising that a mood of optimism prevailed throughout the hemophilia community in the 1970s until AIDS appeared on the horizon, and drastically changed this attitude. The transmission of AIDS to people with hemophilia via the use of their heretofore life-sustaining blood products struck a devastating blow.

As one young man commented, "Hemophilia was something I had all my life, a condition I had continually to adjust to...AIDS is an atom blast overnight."

From the beginning of 1982, the impact of AIDS has been overwhelming. Deep concern and disagreement emerged regarding treatment approaches. The sense of confidence and trust previously enjoyed by the hemophilia community in their health-care providers and blood products was seriously shaken. Patients withheld or reduced their treatments for bleeds, often causing greater pain and disability. The necessary increased vigilance in sterile techniques evoked the self-image of the leper, an untouchable.

The epidemiological link of AIDS with some sexual acts among gay men and shared needle use among intravenous drug users has been particularly distressful to many hemophiliac boys and men. Uncertainties regarding the mode of transmission, as well as the ramifications of being seropositive to the AIDS virus, have created ambivalence and fears about physical closeness, sexual contact, and parenthood.

For some, anxieties about future relationships have caused even greater turmoil. For those who are found to be seropositive (exposed to the AIDS virus and infected with it), although they exhibit no AIDS-related symptoms, the sense of "waiting for the other shoe to drop" can be psychologically devastating.

Also important is the manner in which individuals are told of their antibody status. Individuals diagnosed with ARC (AIDS-related complex) are also extremely vulnerable to psychological distress. Some studies have shown that persons with ARC undergo a greater degree of social and psychological stress than do those actually diagnosed with AIDS. This intense reaction stems in large part from the ambiguity of their condition.

A Diagnosis of AIDS

Due to the life expectancy associated with AIDS, the diagnosis in itself can be devastating. Most people diagnosed with AIDS have not been feeling well for a long time. Prior to diagnosis, they have been extremely anxious and psychologically distressed. Following the actual diagnosis, their worst fears become realized. The most common emotional reactions which accompany the diagnosis include shock, denial, guilt, fear, anger, sadness, bargaining, and acceptance. Patients may be struggling with a flood of conflicting feelings at the time; however, uppermost is their fear of death and dying. Many patients also experience guilt at causing their loved ones undue burdens and suffering. Additionally, there is fear of contagion, loss of self-esteem, fear of loss of physical attractiveness and sexual intimacy, fear of decreased social support and increased dependency, isolation and stigmatization, loss of occupational and financial status, concerns and confusion over options for medical treatment, and an overriding sense of helplessness associated with a degenerative illness.

It is interesting to note that many of these feelings are similar to those often experienced by persons with hemophilia in their response to the challenges of daily living. These emotional reactions may be expressed in very subtle ways. While some people are able to verbalize their fears directly and rationally, others may attempt to strongly deny any concerns, project blame onto others, or displace fears toward other activities or issues. Resentment and anger may be focused on those who are closest, or projected onto homosexuals, health-care providers, or even unto God for "allowing this to happen to me." Increased fatigue, states of tension, confusion, and insecurity may alternate with fierce denial of any problem. Some may adopt an "I don't care" attitude; others may abandon all caution and take dangerous steps.

How to Help

1. Communication and Understanding. Techniques for coping with the anxieties of hemophilia and AIDS vary. Whatever the form of personal coping style, the most important first step is to allow your own feelings to be acknowledged. This holds true for everyone concerned: the patient, his loved ones, and the treatment center staff. Not only is it acceptable to experience conflicting feelings such as helplessness, rage, fear, despair, and deprivation, it is also important to communicate these feelings to someone who instills comfort and trust, and who is able to accept whatever is said. This person may be a loved one, a friend, or a member of the treatment staff who is knowledgeable and sensitive to the emotional turmoil engendered by the diagnosis of AIDS or the fear of contracting or transmitting this disease.

2. Education. Being well-informed about hemophilia and AIDS enables persons with hemophilia to make more appropriate decisions about their treatment and care, as well as any modifications of lifestyle that may be indicated. Individuals should be prepared for questions or comments from fellow workers, school mates, friends, or even family members. Most will be expressions of concern; however, a few may be critical comments arising from people's own fears. Individuals should try to respond with facts based upon valid information so that others may become better informed and less anxious.

3. Risk Behavior Education. People with hemophilia who have been exposed to the AIDS virus, or have been diagnosed with AIDS, can reduce the risk of viral transmission and can improve their health status by adopting the following practices:

a) eat well-balanced meals;

b) get enough rest and exercise;

c) practice good hygiene habits;

d) avoid alcohol and other drugs;

e) do not delay treatment when indicated;

f) observe proper precautions during self-infusion (if blood or concentrate is spilled on the work area, wash the area with 1/4 cup of household liquid bleach, such as Purex, to one quart of water);

g) practice safe sexual behavior by using condoms and by avoiding the exchange of bodily fluids, primarily semen;

h) women exposed to AIDS, or whose sexual partner has been exposed to AIDS, should delay pregnancy until more information about transmission of AIDS to newborns becomes available;

i) maintain close contact with the staff at the treatment center, or the physician, who can explain in greater detail the above recommendations.

Children of Hemophiliacs

If there are children in the family, it is helpful to remember that they, too, are affected by the AIDS crisis, and they are quite perceptive of the feelings of adults close to them. They will become very aware of any marked change in attitude or treatment management practices whether for themselves or their parents. They may also develop involved fantasies from half-veiled remarks by adults around them. Parents should be sensitive to changes in their children's behavior. Particularly significant is withdrawal from activities or friends. Encourage questions and answer them simply and with truthful information at a level of comprehension the child can understand. Parents should be aware that professional advice can be very helpful at this time. Young people with hemophilia may be teased at school or may be asked many questions by their peers regarding their AIDS antibody status or other issues about AIDS. Parents should consider the need for confidentiality of this information and advise their children accordingly.

Parents and children should know that the federal Centers for Disease Control (CDC) as well as the National Hemophilia Foundation support the position that people who are seropositive (i.e., with evidence of previous exposure to the AIDS virus) or who have AIDS or ARC (AIDS-related complex) should be allowed to be in school and in the workplace unless specific circumstances exist which would indicate otherwise.

Resources

Several agencies are available for the person seeking information or help with hemophilia or AIDS-related problems. They offer a variety of services which include:

1) diagnosis and comprehensive treatment;

2) individual and group counseling and psychotherapy;

3) education and information;

4) referrals to community resources;

5) legal representation;

6) insurance information.

Throughout the country, local hemophilia foundations can be an excellent resource. In addition, the National Hemophilia Foundation offers the latest, most accurate information regarding this disease. Local AIDS service providers can also be helpful with AIDS-specific concerns.

Summary

It is not easy having hemophilia, and sometimes life seems totally unfair. The pervasive suffering that AIDS brings to the hemophilia community may make one question the meaning of life itself. However, throughout the years the person with hemophilia and his loved ones have fought to overcome tremendous pain and adversity. Coping with AIDS now becomes the ultimate challenge.

AIDS as a Terminal Illness

Robert W. Krasnow, M.D.

"Because I could not stop for death, he kindly stopped for me," wrote the poet Emily Dickinson. Will death stop for you? I suspect that each person diagnosed with AIDS has wrestled with that prospect. A diagnosis of AIDS easily evokes the possibility—and oftentimes the probability—of death. This wrestling match must surely represent the greatest challenge of having AIDS or any potentially fatal illness. Struggling with death brings into focus a person's past, present, and future—all that was, all that is, and all that might have been. It is a time during which people are most likely to reassess their faith, their beliefs, values, priorities, the meaning of time, and, therefore, of life itself.

Stages of Dying

Elisabeth Kubler-Ross, in her classic book *On Death and Dying*, describes five stages through which dying persons may pass. Dr. Kubler-Ross, a psychiatrist, arrived at these stages through her own in-depth work with terminally ill people. These stages are descriptions of differing psychological states, and are not necessarily experienced in the order given. They may occur separately, simultaneously, in any order, and they may appear, disappear, and reappear. However, they are listed here as Dr. Kubler-Ross listed them.

Shock. These feelings may occur at the first signs of illness, at diagnosis, on being told the illness is incurable or fatal, or anywhere in between. A common response and feeling is "No, not me!" or "It can't be!" The shock may evoke a complete absence of feeling, or emotional numbness. This may be brief, long-lasting, or intermittent.

Denial. Denial can take many forms; it can best be understood by hearing what some people say:

"All this concern, and I'm not really sick."

"AIDS? It's not AIDS. It's just a flare-up of my old hepatitis."

"AIDS! Big deal. I'll probably die in a traffic accident first."

"What do doctors know? I don't plan to change my life one bit."

"The new treatment is going to cure me. . . I'm sure."

Thus, persons with AIDS or other life-threatening illnesses may deny that they are ill at all, that their diagnosis is correct and possibly fatal. They may deny that they are troubled by the diagnosis, or that they will change their lifestyle. They may make unrealistic plans or they may refuse limitations. Denial can come and go; it is often helpful in coping. Denial is only "bad" when self-destructiveness results.

Anger. An individual's feeling may be expressed as "Why me? Why not you? Why not him?" There may be feelings of bitterness and resentment. Anger may be directed at God, doctors, lovers, parents, or a dozen other possible targets. It is often helpful to ventilate anger to someone willing and able to listen.

Bargaining. This response involves feelings like, "Yes, it is me, but. . . I want to live until Christmas," or "until my birthday," or "until my family arrives." It may involve wanting to do a special thing one last time. Most bargains are struck with God, and the bargaining may signal a better ability to face the ultimate facts if they can just be put off a bit.

Depression. This is a familiar feeling for most people. When related to death and dying, it often follows the acknowledgement of *Yes, it is me*—the dealing with the harsh reality of what is happening. Again, it is important to be able to talk with someone who is receptive and sensitive about the sorrow and heartache, someone with whom you can cry comfortably.

Acceptance. Some people reach a point that marks their coming to terms with what is happening, possibly even seeing it as a welcome release. This is not necessarily a goal, and for many people it simply may not happen. Whether or not someone reaches acceptance is neither a good nor a bad reflection on them.

Your Feelings. What will any of us feel in this last portion of our lives? The answer depends largely on a person's present situation, personality, character, temperament, life experiences, and lost hopes and dreams. These will determine how we choose to resolve these feelings.

We have looked at five stages of dying, which include feelings of anger, depression, hopefulness, and calm. A wide range of human emotions may be experienced during this time. Some of these include sadness over past and present losses and those yet to come; anxiety about the unknown, or the known; despair, guilt, shame, outrage, hurt, and even joy. I have listed but a few of the positive emotions, as they are rarely a problem to deal with. The negative emotions, if quite intense, can be disabling and demoralizing.

Help is available when feelings become more than you can cope with. It is important not to adopt an attitude of "How do you expect me to feel?" but rather, "Can I feel better in spite of this?" Using mental health workers, such as psychiatrists, psychologists, social workers, or counselors, who are aware of and sensitive to the psychological and emotional turmoil that accompanies a diagnosis of AIDS, makes sense.

Significant Others

Sometimes it may seem that there is enough for terminally ill persons to do looking after themselves without having to think about others. It will help to remember that those especially close or linked with a person (a lover, spouse, parent, sibling, child, friend) will be undergoing their own complicated reactions to the illness, declining state, and the possibility of death. They, too, may be experiencing some or all of the stages Dr. Kubler-Ross identified, with the consequent denial, anger, bargaining, and depression—and their behavior may be very unpredictable. They may be helpful or negligent, present or absent.

They may be angry about the AIDS or the patient's lifestyle, or they may be very understanding. They may stand by the person or disappear in avoidance. Their reactions may not be as absolute as I have presented; they may resemble instead shades of gray in between. It is likely that their feelings may encompass contradictory emotions similar to those of the patient's.

The terminally ill patient is going to have feelings about these important people's reactions and behavior that may range from hurt and anger to reassurance and gratitude. The patient is certainly entitled to his or her own feelings, but if they become so troublesome that they are having a negative effect on a relationship, it may be wise to seek assistance to work it out. A valued relationship can offer much needed support at this time, and it will be worth the effort to understand and resolve mutual negative feelings rather than rejecting the relationship out of disappointment or anger.

Finishing Life's Business

How devastating it can be to lose control of so many areas of one's life while terminally ill! So many things that might have been done. So much left unsaid and unfinished. Yet this, in large part, is what coming to terms with dying is all about. Since we all die, whether suddenly or after an incapacitating illness, coming to terms with our own dying is part of each of our lives. I am saying that coming to terms with death means coming to terms with life— life that is filled with uncertainty, limitations, thwarted aspirations, and an often abiding sense of incompleteness.

What Can Patients Do for Themselves?

They can gain a sense of control by attending to "real world" concerns, such as wills and property, and by participating in decisions about treatment. They can survey their life to find what has been most pleasant, most meaningful, most fulfilling, and most rewarding. They can avail themselves of the opportunity to bridge some gaps or mend some fences with friends, family, and other significant people. This will help engender a sense of completion, of having made life's circle whole.

Last, and of special importance, is achieving some sense of inner peace and order. This will involve not only acknowledging death's inevitability, but also dealing with long-standing conflicts about oneself and one's life. For example, if a person is gay, it may mean further resolving feelings about homosexuality. It may mean dealing with feelings about career, relationships, family, faith, or the illness itself. This may require the help of a professional, but it is the individual who must provide the willingness and the openness to put life and its meaning in perspective.

The Right to Refuse Treatment

Terminally ill persons have the right to refuse treatment. They may choose not to exercise this right, but it is important for them to know that the choice is theirs. This is a legal right that guarantees us the right to have ultimate control over our own bodies.

In a 1914 decision, Judge Benjamin Cardoza of the New York State Supreme Court declared, "Every human being of adult years and sound mind has a right to determine what shall be done with his own body."

Individuals have the right to refuse treatment regardless of the consequences to themselves; however, if the consequences may be harmful to others, public health laws override this right.

Hospice

"You matter because you are you. You matter to the last moment of your life, and we will do all we can not only to help you die peacefully, but also to [help you] live until you die," wrote Dr. Cicely Saunders, the founder of St. Christopher's Hospice, outside London, in 1967.

During the Middle Ages, hospices were way stations or houses of rest for pilgrims and other weary travelers, as well as for the sick and the dying. In 1967, with the founding of St. Christopher's, the modern hospice movement was born, and today there are hundreds of hospices throughout the western world. Hospice embodies a philosophy of caring for a person with a terminal illness in a way that promises life will end peacefully in a comfortable, caring environment.

What about hospice for you? Currently, hospice home care programs are assisting persons with AIDS to stay at home. Few AIDS patients are utilizing inpatient hospices, primarily because the nature of opportunistic infections requires specialized medical care not usually available in hospice. People usually choose hospice care when curative measures are no longer possible or desirable.

Hospice's great value is in its resurrection of an old belief—that death is a part of life and need not be a time of abandonment of ourselves, our personalities, or our uniqueness. "Living until you die" is the essence of hospice, and as we have choices about how we live, each of us can have choices about how we will die. Hospice encourages tending to those areas of one's life that give it meaning. The opportunity to tie up loose ends, to complete relationships, to reflect on what our having lived has meant to us and others, can offer a sense of harmony and peace at life's end that may have escaped us during life itself.

References

1. Grollman, Earl A. *Concerning Death: A Practical Guide for the Living;* Boston, Beacon Press, 1974.

2. Ogg, Elizabeth. "The Right to Die with Dignity;" Public Affairs Pamphlet No. 587A; New York, Public Affairs Committee, 1983.

3. Sourkes, Barbara M. *The Deepening Shade;* Pittsburgh, University of Pittsburgh Press, 1982.

4. Wilkes, Eric. *The Dying Patient;* Ridgewood, New Jersey, 1982.

An Integrated Approach to Health: Power in the Face of AIDS

Peter Goldblum, Ph.D.

Each day at the AIDS Health Project in San Francisco we are asked, "How can I protect myself from getting AIDS?" With so much information and misinformation available about AIDS and health promotion, sometimes people become confused and overwhelmed. Is the answer vitamins? Should I stop having sex, or maybe I should have more sex? What role does diet play? Is stress really the culprit?

Our answer is simple: Get the best information possible; put it together into a reasonable plan of action; get support for carrying out your health program; and take positive action. We have found that people with a clear and reasonable plan of action are empowered to face the uncertainties of the AIDS crisis. In order to develop a plan of action that has a high likelihood of reducing your risk for AIDS, we suggest that you take a comprehensive view of health and AIDS. By comprehensive we mean a complete view that takes all the important factors into account.

The need for this integrated view of health was brought to light early in our prevention effort. In one of our first health groups, a man with a beautifully muscular body was concerned whether diet and exercise were enough to protect him from getting sick. This man was having many sexual partners in ways we now know to be unsafe. Unfortunately, this man also abused drugs and alcohol, which we know is a major risk factor associated with AIDS. As we talked, he began to understand that he needed to pay attention to the entire array of health factors. Fortunately, this man was able to incorporate these new ideas into a reasonable and comprehensive program. He reduced his unsafe sexual behavior, increased his healthy sexual activities, and began to go to Alcoholics Anonymous for help with his alcohol abuse.

What are the important elements of a comprehensive health plan? The spread of AIDS, like other viral diseases, depends on two things: an agent and a receptive host. Both of these factors need to be considered in your health program. From what we know about HIV (the agent), transmission depends on the interpersonal sharing of bodily fluids, particularly semen and blood. We strongly suspect repeated exposure to the agent increases the risk of AIDS. Therefore, any health program needs to include strategies to reduce exposure to the virus such as the safe-sex guidelines that have been developed by several organizations.

The second part of the health program needs to focus on strengthening your body's defenses against invasion by the virus. We know that not everyone exposed to the virus comes down with AIDS. Again, we suggest an integrated approach to strengthening the immune system. Ask yourself what factors in your life may be affecting your body's ability to protect you from disease. Here are some examples of factors that have been identified to have a negative effect on the immune system: drugs, alcohol, stress, depression, loneliness, and malnutrition.

Making Changes in Health Behavior

Many of you have a fairly clear idea of which health behavior changes would reduce your risk of contracting AIDS. You may have even tried to alter these behavior patterns in the past but failed. Sometimes these failures are due to not seeing the interaction between the behavior you are trying to change and other aspects of your lives. For example, many people find that bar-hopping and pickups are the only ways that they know to meet other sexual partners. If they end this activity, their need to be with others has no way to be fulfilled. This leads to a profound sense of loss. By learning other ways of meeting men or women and having safe sex, certain risky forms of sexual behavior may be averted while still allowing for a healthy social life. In fact, many people have found that they are happier with the new ways of meeting and getting to know others than they were before the AIDS crisis. At the AIDS Health Project, we have developed a three-step process for developing and implementing a health plan which will reduce risk of contracting AIDS and enhance general health.

Step 1: Assess health behavior using an integrated view of health. Determine which changes will have a definite positive effect on preventing AIDS and promoting general health.

Step 2: Develop a health plan.

Step 3: Implement your health plan.

Step 1: Assessing Health Behavior

The first step in assessing one's health behavior is to get a clear picture of one's current health practices. Taking an integrated approach, it is important to review various health factors. Here are some areas we suggest:

Sexual Activity. What is your level of risk for exposure to the AIDS virus? Compare your sexual activities to those listed in the widely distributed safe-sex guidelines. (See Section Five; "Safe-Sex Guidelines") What kinds of sex are you having, how many different partners do you have, and what is the status of their health?

Drugs and Alcohol. Evidence suggests that this is a very important risk factor for AIDS. Anyone sharing IV-drug needles needs to stop. Drugs and alcohol cause stress on the immune system which may reduce its functioning. Alcohol and drugs alter one's judgment, which may make one more prone to engage in higher risk sexual activities. Are drugs and alcohol a problem for you?

Stress. Stress is the psycho-physiological response to change. Stress results when people perceive an imbalance in their lives between the demands placed on them and the resources that they have available to meet these demands. Since high levels of stress over an extended period of time can negatively affect the immune system, reducing one's stress is important. By restructuring aspects of our lives, we may prevent harmful stress. There are also ways to reduce the effects of stress, primarily by learning various forms of relaxation. What is your level of stress? How are you coping with stress?

Social Support. Spouses, friends, lovers, and family members can be part of the problem or part of the solution to life's problems. How much support do you have in your life? How fulfilling are your relationships?

Nutrition and Exercise. Although few of us are malnourished, there is some evidence that attention to our diets will improve our general health. Also, some foods may cause stress, for example, caffeine, chocolate, and sugar. Exercise has been shown to reduce stress, improve our emotional outlook, and be an important aspect of general health management.

Attitudes and Self-Concept. Our general outlook and the way we feel may affect our health. In times of crisis, old negative beliefs about yourself may re-emerge. Feelings of hopelessness and helplessness may pervade your consciousness. These feelings should not be confused with appropriate feelings of sadness, anger, or disappointment which we all experience. What is the emotional tone of your life now? How are you coping with feelings related to the AIDS crisis? Once you have identified the areas in which you need to make changes, be specific about what specifically you need to change. Change means action. How willing are you to let go of some behavior patterns that no longer work for you, while adding new constructive ones to your life?

Step 2: Develop a Health Plan

Developing a health plan means setting a behavioral goal and developing a strategy for reaching your goal. A goal is a specific behavior which can be observed and measured. For example, "I will reduce my alcohol consumption to two drinks per week."

Note that the behavioral goal is very specific. It tells you exactly what you need to do. You can also determine later whether you met your goal or not. We have found that a good deal of time is needed to fine tune one's goals. Sometimes people try to accomplish too much at first. What is important is to select a goal which is meaningful to you.

Ask yourself: "What change in health behavior will most affect my chances of preventing AIDS? What do I do now which most endangers my health?" Selecting a strategy which will bring about the results you seek is another aspect of developing your health plan. As the old saying goes, "There's more than one way to skin a cat."

Here are some hints:

1) What has worked for you in the past?

2) What is your change style—"cold turkey" or "slowly but surely?"

3) What approaches best suit the type of behavior you are trying to change? For example, you would use a different strategy to learn how to meet new sex partners than you would to stop sharing IV needles.

4) Be honest. If you fool anyone, it's only yourself.

5) Get feedback. Check out with your friends what you're doing.

6) Take responsibility. In the final analysis, the decision is yours.

Step 3: Implementing the Health Plan

One of the techniques we encourage members in our workshops to use is behavior contracts. This is merely an agreement that a person makes with himself, and perhaps with another person, to make certain changes. The contract includes the agreement and consequences. An agreement is the behavioral goal. It includes both the behavior and time interval. For example, "I will give one massage and receive one massage each week." Set up consequences in advance: "What will happen if I keep my agreement, or if I do not live up to my agreement?" We sometimes call these "reinforcers."

Many people we have talked with find that giving themselves a reward is quite difficult. This takes some practice. In regard to consequences, identify things or events which you enjoy. Be sure they are things which you have control over, such as taking yourself to the movies, getting a massage, or buying yourself a new shirt. Get friends to help you with this.

An important aspect of any behavioral change project is to re-evaluate from time to time to determine if the project is working. If it is not, then you need to change it.

Facing AIDS Together

A crisis can bring out the best in us. In our groups we have frequently seen the beauty of people reaching out to each other. Some of the most powerful and loving moments are moments of confrontation. The message is always the same. "I care too much about you to keep quiet. You're putting yourself in danger by what you're doing. Please stop."

Making changes isn't easy. It need not be lonely. We encourage you to include others both in your health plan and in helping to make it work. If we can find the courage to face this crisis directly, the power that we achieve as individuals and as a community in facing this terrible disease can enrich our lives.

Section Three

A Medical Perspective

HIV (AIDS virus) is transmitted by intimate sexual contact with exchange of genital secretions....It is also transmitted by blood contamination, by which we do not mean a splash onto the skin or mucous membranes. It is most likely blood into the bloodstream, such as the way IV-drug users (who share needles) inject into their bloodstream blood that remains in the syringe from the prior shooter, or the way hemophiliacs get factor VIII, or others get blood transfusions directly into the vein. It is blood to bloodstream, not blood onto a laboratory bench or onto a toilet seat.

"AIDS: A Medical Overview"

AIDS: A Medical Overview
The Antibody Test
AIDS Defined Illnesses
Coping with ARC
Medical Impact of AIDS on Hemophilia

AIDS: A Medical Overview

Donald Abrams, M.D.

What exactly is this disease that is making such waves in the United States and the world? Has there been anything like it in the history of medicine? AIDS is described by the Centers for Disease Control (CDC) in Atlanta as "the presence of a reliably diagnosed disease that is at least moderately indicative of a problem of underlying cellular immune deficiency in people less than the age of sixty who have no other known causes of immune deficiency, are not on any immune suppressant therapy, and do not have a lymphoma or Hodgkin's disease, both known to be associated with immune suppression." This is pretty vague. What is really meant?

AIDS is an infection of the white blood cell called the lymphocyte, the building block of the immune system, by a virus. This virus, a new virus, has been given a new name: HIV (human immunodeficiency virus). This name clarifies a lot of things muddled by prior names given the virus. It tells us who the virus infects: humans. It tells us what it causes: immunodeficiency or breakdown in the immune system. So HIV is the new name of this new virus which

This overview of the epidemiology and immunology of AIDS was prepared for a conference, "Comprehensive Care of the AIDS Patient: A Workshop," which was held in San Francisco, September 1986. It formerly appeared in *California Nursing Review*, Vol.53, October 1986. Reprinted with permission.

infects predominantly the white blood cell, the lymphocyte, the building block of our immune system. In so doing, it leads to a variety of so-called opportunistic infections and unusual malignancies.

THE IMMUNE SYSTEM

I. The Players

To understand the clinical diseases we see in AIDS and how they can result from infection with this new virus, some background information on the normal human immune system is helpful. The building block of the immune system is the lymphocyte, a white blood cell. Looking under the microscope, we can clearly distinguish which white blood cells are lymphocytes from those which are the polys. The polys, so-called because of the many segments of their nucleus, are there to promote wound healing and to fight bacterial infections. Lymphocytes fight viral infections and intracellular infections.

The immune system of humans is made up of groups of these lymphocytes which form lymph nodes. These nodes are scattered throughout the body, but are normally not palpable on physical examination of healthy people. The thymus is a gland over which lies the heart. The thymus programs a subset of lymphocytes called the T-cells. The thymus is an organ which shrinks and essentially disappears by the time we are five years old, but continues to secrete hormones that take care of programming these T-cells. B-cells are the other form of lymphocytes made in the bone marrow.

II. The Function of the Immune System Components

The spleen acts like a big lymph node and contains T-cells, B-cells, and another white blood cell, which is known as a monocyte when it is in the bloodstream, but a macrophage when it goes into the tissues. All of these cells have different functions in protecting our body. The immune system is there to protect us against foreign invaders, usually micro-organisms. When the body sees a protein—for example, an organism which does not belong to the body—it is usually ingested by the scavenger cell or the macrophage. Then it is presented to either the T-cell or the B-cell. B-cells work by secreting a protein into the bloodstream, an antibody, that goes out and neutralizes the infectious agent. B-cells themselves do not go out and eat up the organism, but they secrete the antibody into circulation. This is called *humoral immunity* because B-cells make a humor or substance that goes into our plasma. On the other hand,

T-cells work not by secreting a protein, but by the cell itself going out and ingesting the invading protein or organism. T-cells are responsible for what is called *cell-mediated immunity,* because it is the actual cell itself, the lymphocyte, that does all the work.

Sometimes, B-cells go wrong, and instead of making antibodies to hepatitis, herpes, or the AIDS virus, they get confused and make antibodies to parts of our own body. The classical disease for this is lupus, a disease of young women, where the body makes antibodies to its own nuclei, the DNA in the body. This phenomenon, where B-cells get confused and make antibodies against one's own body, is called auto-immunity.

All these immune system cells originally come from the bone marrow. B-cells mature into plasma cells and secrete the immunoglobulins which are of various subclasses; IgG is the most familiar immunoglobulin subclass. T-cells go through the thymus where they get programmed to perform their function. Their most important job with regard to AIDS is killing virally infected cells and tumor-cells. It is felt that all of us at any given moment have a few cells which are becoming malignant and have the potential of becoming a cancer or a tumor, but because we have healthy functioning T-cells, those cells are eradicated before they can ever grow to tumor proportions.

In the T-cell category there are two families: the helper T-cells and the suppressor T-cells. They do pretty much what their names suggest. Helper T-cells are there to boost and augment the function of the whole immune system; they can be thought of as the orchestra conductor of the coordinated immune response. They work on the monocyte-macrophage and on the B-cell, telling it to secrete immunoglobulins to protect the body from this infection. Suppressor cells are not bad or evil; they are there to turn off the immune response when the job is done. Normally, healthy people have twice as many of these helper cells in their bloodstream as they have suppressor cells. Looking under the microscope at a blood sample, one cannot determine which of the lymphocytes are B-cells or T-cells—which are helper cells or which are suppressor cells. Sophisticated monoclonal antibodies that fluoresce help distinguish these cells into the different categories. Again, the important thing to remember is that healthy individuals have a ratio of helper cells to suppressor cells of 2:1.

III. The Immune System Changes in AIDS

In our patients with AIDS and opportunistic infections the situation is exactly reversed. What makes the ratio abnormal is that patients with AIDS have a marked decrease in the number of their helper cells. Those patients with the most severe manifestations of AIDS, opportunistic infections, have twice as many suppressors as helpers. Patients with Kaposi's sarcoma or the lymph node problem have an equalization: the same number of helper and suppressor cells, again caused by a decrease in the helper cell population. We noted early in the epidemic that apparently healthy homosexual men had abnormal helper/suppressor ratios compared to healthy heterosexuals. This was disturbing. In different cities there were different percentages of the population affected. We now know this really reflects how many of them had been infected with the AIDS virus.

In addition to having this abnormal ratio with the decrease in their helper T-cells, most AIDS patients have too much immunoglobulin. Their B-cells are hyperactive; they are turned on and are squirting out these antibodies for protection. AIDS is not really a total immune deficiency, because the B-cells are turned on and the T-cells are decreased. What we have is an immune imbalance or dysfunction. In the next section we will explore the cause of this immune dysfunction.

THE AIDS VIRUS

From the very beginning, many investigators thought AIDS must be caused by a virus. We knew from prior experience that viruses can affect the immune system. If a skin test is placed for tuberculosis in someone who had been positive in the past and has a viral infection at the time of the test, the result may be negative. The cellular immune system which is responsible for skin-test reactivity is gone. In other words, people do not respond positively to skin tests when they have a viral infection. Most viral infections which cause imbalances of immune regulation usually cause very transient or short-lived immune dysfunction. We knew early on that different viruses caused immune imbalances very similar to what we see in AIDS. Two viruses in the herpes family, cytomegalovirus and Epstein-Barr, both cause a form of mononucleosis. They also cause an increase in the suppressor cells and a decrease in the helper cells, and turn on immunoglobulin production. However, when we looked at antibodies to cytomegalovirus or Epstein-Barr virus in AIDS patients and in risk group controls, we found that 100 percent of the gay men tested in San Francisco—whether they had AIDS or did not—had antibodies to those two viruses. This suggested that neither CMV nor EBV could be seriously considered as a cause of this disease.

I. The Announcement

It was not until April 1984 that we became convinced we were closing in on the cause of the disease. Actually, it was in 1983 that a group from the Pasteur Institute in Paris first reported their finding of a new virus. They took a lymph node from a patient with the AIDS-related lymphadenopathy syndrome, and cultured an unusual virus called "lymphadenopathy-associated virus," or LAV. They sent some of the virus, which was in a family called retroviruses, to Dr. Robert Gallo's laboratory in Bethesda. Dr. Gallo was known as an expert in retrovirology. Retroviruses, although they are not new viruses in the history of the world, were only first discovered to cause diseases in humans in 1979–1980 by Dr. Gallo; also by a group of Japanese investigators who defined human T-cell leukemia-lymphoma virus type I (HTLV-I), a retrovirus that causes an aggressive form of lymphoma. Dr. Gallo was able to isolate a similar virus from AIDS patients in the U.S. We now know that the AIDS virus not only infects the immune system, but also infects the central nervous system. It may have been originally miscategorized by putting it in the human T-cell lymphoma-leukemia virus family. That is why we have now moved toward the human immunodeficiency virus (HIV) name.

II. What Is a Retrovirus?

What is a retrovirus? Why is this virus such a particularly difficult virus to combat? A virus is simply a piece of genetic information, either DNA or RNA, surrounded by a protein coat to protect it from the environment. A retrovirus is a single piece of RNA surrounded by a protein coat, or envelope. Normally the flow of genetic information in life is from DNA, which codes for a piece of RNA which in turn codes for a protein. A unique enzyme allows this retrovirus, a piece of RNA, to go backwards against the flow of life (hence a "retro"virus) and make itself into a piece of DNA. The virus DNA then gets inserted into the DNA in the nucleus of the cell that it infects, and it stays there for the life of the cell.

III. Who Has the Virus?

In culturing people with AIDS and people with AIDS-related complex (ARC) for the virus, the results are rather interesting. When we actually try to culture the virus from people with AIDS, it is more difficult to culture than from patients with ARC, the earlier or milder stages of the disease. Why is that? The virus infects the immune system, leading to its destruction. Those white blood cells which are the building blocks of the immune system get destroyed by the virus infection. So by the time we take blood from an AIDS patient to see if we can culture the virus, he may not have any more of those white blood cells—no more home for the virus. So he would be less likely to be shedding the virus than patients who have the earlier or less severe manifestations of the disease.

IV. Where Is the Virus?

Which secretions have HIV? Because it is an infection of the white blood cell, the lymphocyte, it is no surprise the virus is found in the blood, in the bone marrow where the blood is made, and in the lymph nodes where the lymphocytes reside. The virus could also be found within cells in the plasma. Similarly, the virus has been isolated from saliva, urine, semen, and cervical secretions. The richest sources of HIV are semen and blood. In semen, it is not sperm itself that is infected. Each ejaculation contains about 2,000,000 lymphocytes, the white blood cells which contain the virus, and these likely transmit the virus. Cervical and vaginal secretions also contain the virus, but in a very low percentage of women who are positive for the antibodies.

Most of the fear has centered around the issue of saliva. Can saliva transmit the disease? Probably not. Only a small percentage of infected people actually harbor the virus in the saliva. If HIV were easily transmitted by the saliva, the epidemic would be more widespread and would have affected more people outside of the known risk groups. The weight of current evidence speaks against salivary transmission.

The AIDS virus can also be found in tears. Certainly, not too many diseases known are transmitted by tears. It is difficult to imagine how tears could transmit a disease except to opthalmologists, perhaps. Should eye doctors be concerned that they may next be a potential risk group for developing AIDS? Again, looking at the epidemiology of the disease, we see that eye doctors in San Francisco are not developing AIDS. Tears are probably not an effective source of transmission. Seriously, although the virus may eventually be detected in probably every body fluid, including perspiration, it is not likely to be able to transmit the disease.

HIV is *transmitted by intimate sexual contact with exchange of genital secretions*—that is, semen and probably vaginal cervical secretions. It is also *transmitted by blood contamination,* by which we do not mean an occasional splash onto the skin or mucous membranes. It is most likely blood into the bloodstream such as the way IV-drug users inject blood into their blood stream that remains in the syringe from the prior shooter, or the way hemophiliacs get factor VIII or others get blood transfusions directly into the vein. It is blood to bloodstream, not blood onto a laboratory bench or onto a toilet seat. If it were that easily spread, there would be millions more infection cases than we detect right now. Intimate sexual contact, with exchange of genital secretions, and blood contamination are the two routes of transmission of HIV and, therefore, AIDS.

V. Who Gets AIDS?

Homosexual and Bisexual Men. The first cases of AIDS were reported in July 1981 in the Centers for Disease Control's *Morbidity and Mortality Weekly Report.* At that time, ten patients were reported with pneumocystis carinii pneumonia, a rare lung infection, and twenty-two patients with Kaposi's sarcoma, an ususual skin cancer. Of these first cases, 95 percent were homosexual or bisexual men. Shortly thereafter in 1981–1982, other risk groups became apparent. Since the beginning of the epidemic, 27 percent of all cases have been diagnosed in heterosexuals. These heterosexuals, however, have belonged to well-defined risk groups. The gay and bisexual male groups continue to account for about 70 percent of all AIDS diagnosed in the U.S. These numbers are changing as more and more heterosexuals contract AIDS. Somehow, we need to ascertain what percentage of the disease is in homosexual men and what percentage of the disease is in bisexual men. Gay men have sex with other gay men. Bisexual men have sex with both men and women. If we are concerned about potential spread of the disease in all members of the population, it is also the bisexual male group that needs to be educated.

Intravenous Drug Users. Other than homosexual or bisexual men, the first group noted to be at risk for AIDS were the intravenous drug users. These were men or women who used intravenous drugs—usually heroin, but also cocaine or speed. Here was the first instance in which women were found to be as likely as men to be infected with the virus.

Racial distribution of AIDS in the U.S. reveals about two-thirds of all patients are Caucasian. In the intravenous drug using group, the disease is predominantly one of the minority population with about 66 percent of the people in this group being black or Hispanic. Interestingly, Asians (gay or not) currently seem to be free of the problem of AIDS. Although there is a large Asian homosexual community in San Francisco, there have been very few reported cases of AIDS. In Japan, a very populous country, only sixteen cases of AIDS have been reported—half of them in hemophiliacs, half in homosexual men.

The Haitian Problem. The third group noted to be at increased risk to develop the disease is actually no longer listed by the Centers for Disease Control as an official AIDS risk group. In 1981–1982, it was noticed that Haitian immigrants to the United States—especially in Miami, Brooklyn, and the Bronx—were developing AIDS with increased frequency compared to the general population. Overall, Haitian immigrants to the U.S. account for three to four percent of all the AIDS cases reported. However they are no longer included as a separate risk group and are counted in the "other" or "unknown" category. Why is this? Former President for Life Duvalier of Haiti, before he left office, managed to convince the Centers for Disease Control that being Haitian was not in itself a risk factor for developing AIDS. Pointing out that such a fallacy compares to saying San Franciscans are at risk for developing AIDS, he asked the CDC to please look more carefully at the reasons why the Haitians who were getting AIDS, both the immigrants to the United States and those in Haiti, were developing the disease. What was the real risk factor? This resulted in the CDC removing Haitians from the list of known risk groups and listing Haitian immigrants to the United States in the "other" or "unknown" categories.

Investigators visiting Haiti have, in fact, reported a remarkable epidemic of the disease in this island nation. Sharing the island Hispanola with the Dominican Republic, Haiti is currently having a pronounced epidemic of AIDS, while the Dominican Republic has only a few isolated cases on the northern and southern shores, thought to be a result of what we call "sexual tourism." Why Haiti is in the midst of an epidemic very similar to ours is unclear at this time.

Hemophiliacs and Transfusion Recipients. The fourth group noted to be at risk to develop AIDS were men who had hemophilia, which is a congenital bleeding disorder due to a lack of factor VIII. To prevent themselves from bleeding, hemophiliacs intermittently transfuse themselves with factor VIII concentrate, each unit of which is comprised of blood donated by 20 to 20,000 blood donors. While hemophiliacs normally die of bleeding complications, 1981–1982 saw an increase in the number of hemophiliacs suffering from pneumocystis pneumonia. It then became clear that they had the same underlying immune problem as people with AIDS. This was the first revelation that the disease could be transmitted through contaminated blood products. Since the onset of the epidemic, three percent of AIDS patients have developed the disease through contaminated blood products—either hemophiliacs transfusing factor VIII, or people who have received other transfused blood products (usually packed red cells or platelets).

Heterosexual Transmission and the African Experience. A very small number of AIDS cases in the United States have been transmitted through heterosexual sexual contact, although the actual number of cases climb as the epidemic increases. These are women who have had sex with bisexual men, IV-drug users, hemophiliacs or transfusion recipients, or men who have had sex with women in these risk groups who have been infected with the virus. Actually, now that we know AIDS is a sexually transmitted disease caused by a virus, this makes sense. Viruses do not know whether they infect man or woman, heterosexual or homosexual. So if the disease is in the population, and if unprotected, widespread sexual activity is occurring, there is no reason to be surprised that the virus is transmitted through heterosexual sexual activity.

We learn a lot by looking at the situation which is currently unfolding in central Africa. Some of the first cases of AIDS to appear were actually in women, European women, who had lived in central Africa. One of the first reported cases was a woman who had been a surgeon in Zaire and who became ill with AIDS when she returned home to Denmark in 1976. In Brussels, in 1981 and 1982, a number of black Africans returned from the central part of that continent with a disease that was very similar to what we were calling AIDS in the United States. Zaire and Rwanda are the former Belgium Congo. People who become sick there sometimes travel back to Brussels to obtain health care. With the increasing number of AIDS cases being seen in Belgium, a group of investigators went from the World Health Organization, the CDC, and Brussels down to Kinshasa, the main city in Zaire. They found that large numbers of adults hospitalized in Kinshasa had AIDS. Current suppression of information about AIDS in Africa prevents us from viewing the full extent of the problem.

In 1985, at the First International Conference on AIDS, in Atlanta, there were suggestions that AIDS in Africa was a bit of a problem. In 1986, at the Second International Conference on AIDS, in Paris, a lot of attention was devoted to the problem of AIDS in Africa. Six percent of the adults in Zaire are found to have the AIDS virus antibody, and 18 percent of the blood donors in Rwanda have the antibody to the AIDS virus. The incidence is generally higher in the cities compared to the rural areas. The incidence in African prostitutes can be as high as 88 percent in some countries. In Africa, another difference is seen; the disease is constituted of about 50 percent men and 50 percent women. In the United States, currently 92 percent of all AIDS cases are in men and 8 percent in women. In Africa, it is quite clear that the disease spreads through heterosexual contact, both from man to woman and vice-versa.

Does the African situation mean that we can expect this 50–50 male to female ratio in the United States? At a recent Public Health Service conference, it was predicted that the heterosexual spread of AIDS in the United States will only account for about 4.5 percent of all AIDS in 1991. Again, hepatitis B is found in IV-drug users, homosexual men, and people who have many blood transfusions. Hepatitis B in the United States has not become the epidemic venereal disease in the heterosexual community. In Africa, however, it is. In Africa, 20 percent of all people have antibodies to the hepatitis B virus. The point is that we cannot take the situation in a developing country and extrapolate it to the situation that may eventually occur in the United States or other industrialized nations, because viral infections can have different pictures or different epidemiology in different parts of the world.

Pediatric AIDS. Another group of AIDS patients receiving a lot of attention is the small number of children who have been diagnosed with the disease. Compared to the over 20,000 adults, only 289 children have been diagnosed as of May 1986. The critical point here is how the children got the disease. And it's no mystery. The children with AIDS were predominantly born to mothers who were in a risk group: intravenous drug-using women or women of Haitian extraction. The disease-causing virus is passed from the mother to the child inside the womb. Another 20 percent of AIDS in children is caused by another known route of transmission: *contaminated blood products*. AIDS has developed in infants requiring blood transfusions at birth as well as in children with hemophilia or other coagulation disorders. Therefore, 95 percent of the AIDS in children is explainable. Only 5 percent of infected children belong to "other" or "unknown" categories of risk.

Numerous studies have analyzed children living in the homes of adults who had AIDS. None of these children has developed AIDS. None of these children has made antibodies to the virus. A large study comprised of 100 children living in homes of AIDS patients demonstrated that none of them had antibodies to the virus; none of them has the disease. Similarly, there is concern about children being together with other children. Institutionalized children in Europe have also been evaluated. Some of the children had antibodies to the AIDS virus because they were hemophiliacs. They were also in an orphanage together. Children in that setting do what children everywhere do: they scratch, they bite, they play with each other's feces, etc. None of the other children had antibodies to the virus. None of the other children contracted the disease. Similar to adults, AIDS transmission in children occurs by known routes. AIDS in children develops predominantly by transmission from the mother and also through contaminated blood products. AIDS is not transmitted in children, or adults, by way of casual contact. However, we continue to face hysteria and fear of AIDS in schools. Hopefully, as knowledge of the lack of risk in this situation becomes disseminated, people will become much less hysterical and much more rational about the disease.

The Origin of AIDS

Where did the virus come from in the first place? More and more evidence is suggesting that the African green monkey may be the link in the AIDS mystery. In Africa, many animals have been tested to see if they have any viruses in their bloodstreams similar to the AIDS virus. When gibbons, gorillas, and baboons were studied, none was positive for antibodies to the AIDS virus. However, in the African green monkey 40 percent had antibodies to a virus that was very similar to the human AIDS virus. The French recently reported a new AIDS-like virus they found in people from an island off the west coast of Africa, which partially cross reacts with the human AIDS virus and partially reacts with the monkey AIDS virus. It is like a hybrid virus. Possibly what could have happened is that a virus which had been infecting monkeys for a long time, with or without causing disease, somehow got out of the monkey population and into the human population where it had never before been seen. Any time you introduce a new virus to a human population, like measles to Hawaiians, the effect can be devastating. This could be what is happening with the AIDS virus. It has been postulated that the virus got out of the animal population in the early '70s in Africa. With the great industrialization, centralization, and urbanization occurring in that continent during the past ten years, the virus infection has been amplified and intensified, leading to the current problems that exist worldwide.

The Antibody Test

Jennifer Lang, R.N., M.N., and Ronald Mitsuyasu, M.D.

With the discovery of the AIDS retrovirus (HIV) came the antibody test, which allowed us to detect the presence of antibodies to the virus. This test does not detect the virus itself, but rather the antibodies to the virus in people who have been infected. Nearly 100 percent of patients with AIDS are found to have antibody evidence of infection with the virus, which is logical when saying that this virus *causes* the disease. Patients with the AIDS-related complex (ARC) have about a 95 percent rate of positivity for antibodies to the virus. The incidence of antibodies to the AIDS virus in healthy heterosexual populations is very low. In a blood donor group, it's felt to be .04 percent; that is, 4 out of every 10,000 healthy heterosexuals will show evidence of antibodies to the virus. The incidence in the healthy gay male population is variable depending on where you look. In San Francisco, it is about 50 percent. In cities like Stockholm, Sweden, it is about 10 percent. In Chicago it might be 35 percent. The incidence in intravenous drug users is also dependent on geographical location. In Newark and New York City, 75 to 80 percent of intravenous drug users have antibodies to the AIDS virus, meaning that they have been infected with the AIDS virus at some point. Fortunately, in San Francisco, only 10 to 20 percent of intravenous drug users have antibodies to the virus at this time, no doubt explaining why San Francisco has not yet seen a large number of

AIDS cases in the IV-drug using community. However, in 1979 or 1980 the incidence of antibody positivity in the gay community was also 10 to 20 percent. So, if something is not done to stop the spread of HIV in the IV-drug using community, it could also become a big major problem here.

Blood Banking

What is the "AIDS test" that is done in blood banks? It is simply a test for the AIDS antibody. The method used is called an "enzyme-linked immunoabsorbent assay" (ELISA). In general it is a very good test. To put it simply, we stick the AIDS virus at the bottom of a test well, adding serum for testing antibodies to the virus. If there is an antibody to the virus, it will stick to the virus because they interlock. Then the well is washed. Another antibody made in a goat recognizes human antibody. So if the blood specimen being tested had an antibody to the AIDS virus, this goat antibody will stick to the human antibody. Attached to the goat antibody is an enzyme. When the substrate of that enzyme is added to the well, a color change occurs. A spectrophotometer reads the color change, produces a value which is then scored as either positive or negative.

There are a number of places where there might be some error, but in general, the test is 99 percent accurate. That means 1 percent are going to be inaccurate. If a hundred people go to the blood bank, one person is going to be told, "Your blood test is positive; you have antibodies to the AIDS virus," but they do not. That is called a false positive. These are not bad odds if we miss only one person in a hundred. So we discard one unit of blood. However, in the United States, each year 11 million people donate a unit of blood. So one percent of those is 110,000 units of blood that need to be discarded because they are read as positive for the AIDS virus, even though, in fact, they are not. Regardless of the uncertainty this information implies, 110,000 people must be told they have been infected with the AIDS virus—even though this is not true.

To avoid these false positives, we do what is called a "confirmatory test." The western blot is another technique available for detecting antibodies to the AIDS virus. The virus is disrupted with a detergent. Electricity is run through to divide it into different molecular weight components. Then, the serum being tested for antibodies is added. After a few more stages, the different molecular weight components can be seen if the blots are positive. This western blot should be done on people not in a known AIDS risk group who come up with a positive ELISA test. Women seem more likely to have false positive results.

Initially, blood banks became concerned that once they instituted ELISA testing, many people from the AIDS risk groups would come to the blood banks to donate blood just to find out if they were positive or negative. This does not consider the intelligence or the beneficence of people in risk groups to assume they would intentionally contaminate the blood supply merely to find out their own results. To avoid this, the state established alternative test sites where people can go—completely anonymously and with confidentiality assured—and have their blood tested to determine if they are positive or negative for antibodies to the AIDS virus. This is certainly better than having people donate to the blood bank, for a number of reasons. First of all, just as there are false positives, there are also false negatives. That means somebody who is really positive may be called negative in the ELISA test. Similarly, an antibody to a virus is made shortly after infection, but not immediately. So some people may have the actual virus in their blood, but not have an antibody until some time later. This recently occurred when a man in Colorado donated blood shortly after having a sexual encounter. His blood was negative for the AIDS antibody, but he did have the virus. The recipient of his blood became infected.

Why isn't it good to have an antibody? Doesn't that protect us from the virus? We have mentioned hepatitis a few times already. If somebody has the hepatitis B virus in their blood stream, they do not have an antibody to the virus. Only when the virus itself goes away does the antibody come. Then that antibody protects the people from getting hepatitis B again. Once you've had it, that's it. A different situation exists with herpes simplex, the virus that causes cold sores. All of us probably have antibodies to that virus by the time we reach our teens. However, we continue to get cold sores throughout our lives, because the *herpes antibody is nonprotective*. Similarly in AIDS, a high percentage of people who have the antibody, may also have the virus. Especially people with the AIDS-related complex (ARC) may have both the antibody and the virus existing together. We all know that antibodies do not transmit disease. So why is the blood bank looking for antibodies to the virus? In the absence of actually trying to culture each unit of blood for the AIDS virus, doing an antibody test is a pretty good way to simultaneously eliminate blood that may also have the virus.

The Meaning of a Positive Test

Although the antibody test may be useful in the blood bank, is it of value in testing people? Again, it isn't the antibodies to the virus that cause the disease. At this time, we do not know the natural history of people who are antibody positive. We don't know if all of them are going to get AIDS twenty years down the line, or if some of them will never have any problem again and just always remain positive to the antibody. It is the virus which causes disease. And the disease is diagnosed clinically, quite easily, without necessarily obtaining a blood test for antibodies. AIDS is a clinical diagnosis. A positive antibody test is not a diagnosis of AIDS.

AIDS Defined Illnesses

Jennifer Lang, M.N., R.N., and Ronald Mitsuyasu, M.D.

I. OPPORTUNISTIC INFECTIONS

Opportunistic infections are caused by organisms which commonly occur in the environment; persons with a normally functioning immune system have a natural resistance to these organisms. Only when someone's immune system is suppressed can these viruses, fungi, protozoa, and mycobacteria seize the "opportunity" to cause infection. Therefore, people with AIDS are at risk of developing opportunistic infections, which can be frequent and serious. The organisms causing opportunistic infections are listed here.

Viruses

The viral infections most commonly seen in persons with AIDS are caused by members of the herpes virus family. Cytomegalovirus (CMV), Epstein-Barr virus (EBV), herpes simplex I (cold sores), herpes simplex II (genital herpes), and herpes zoster (shingles) are all seen frequently. Both CMV and EBV cause infectious mononucleosis-like illnesses with fevers, sweats, loss of appetite, sore throat, lymphadenopathy (swollen lymph nodes), and severe fatigue of several weeks' duration.

Occasionally, an infection can occur without any symptoms. Both CMV and EBV can be transmitted in urine, saliva, sputum, and semen. Commonly called "the kissing disease," these infections are very common in all segments of the population, but even more so among gay men. Both CMV and EBV are known as chronic viruses which remain dormant in the body after an initial infection and then are capable of reactivating during periods of immunosuppression. Most, if not all, persons with AIDS demonstrate active infections with CMV and EBV alone or together during the course of AIDS. In the immunosuppressed person with AIDS, CMV may be the cause of pneumonia, gastrointestinal symptoms (vomiting and diarrhea), hepatitis, or impaired vision.

When herpes simplex I and II appear with AIDS, the symptoms are different for people with AIDS than for people with normally functioning immune systems. The herpes sores may last longer, they may be more difficult to heal, and they may be more likely to spread to other locations. Herpes zoster (shingles) occurs as a result of reactivation of an old chickenpox virus which has been dormant along the lining of a nerve since childhood. Although frequently seen in older people who do not have AIDS, the shingles seen with AIDS takes longer to heal, is more likely to spread, and may require hospital treatment with an antiviral drug.

Fungi

Candida and cryptococcus are two fungi frequently seen in people with AIDS. Candida is very commonly found on the mucous membranes of the mouth and vagina. In AIDS, candida overgrows on the mucous membranes of the mouth, gastrointestinal tract, and sometimes in internal organs. When infecting the mouth, it is known as thrush and is associated with visible creamy white patches, reddened mucous membranes, and some discomfort in chewing and swallowing. Cryptococcus neoformans is a fungus which is inhaled into the lungs, but most commonly it infects the lining of the brain causing headaches, blurred vision, confusion, depression, uncontrolled excitement, and inappropriate speech.

Protozoa

The protozoans pneumocystis carinii, cryptosporidia, and toxoplasma gondii are responsible for three major opportunistic infections. Pneumocystis carinii causes a pneumonia which develops slowly and is not easily recognized in its early stages. Pneumocystis carinii pneumonia (PCP) is the most common of all the opportunistic infections.

Cryptosporidiosis is the name given to a diarrheal infection caused by the protozoan cryptosporidia. This organism attaches itself to the lining of the small and large intestines and prevents absorption of nutrients. The diarrhea is severe with frequent watery stools and abdominal cramping.

Toxoplasmosis, transmitted hand to mouth primarily from cat feces, is a common infection with very few symptoms in most segments of the population. In AIDS, toxoplasmosis tends to be more severe, causing an inflammation of the brain with fevers, changes in ability to move, and personality or behavior changes.

Mycobacteria

The most commonly known member of this family, m. tuberculosis, which causes lung tuberculosis, is sometimes seen in persons with AIDS. More frequently, mycobacterium avium-intracellulare (MAI) is seen, infecting the bloodstream, internal organs, bone marrow, and lymph nodes, but rarely the lungs. The most common symptom is fever. Persons with normal immune system function are not at risk of developing MAI.

II. KAPOSI'S SARCOMA

Epidemic vs. Classical

Kaposi's sarcoma, one of the opportunistic conditions seen in AIDS, is not a new cancer. On the contrary, it has been known to exist in a classic, non-fatal form for over a century and is found in another form in parts of Africa. This section will discuss Kaposi's sarcoma as it appears in its classic European origin, endemic African framework, and most recently, AIDS-related epidemic form.

Classical: Kaposi's sarcoma was first described over a century ago by the Hungarian dermatologist, Moricz Kaposi, as a slow-growing tumor affecting primarily elderly men of Ashkenazi Jewish or Mediterranean origin. Although the term sarcoma (which means soft tissue tumor) is used, this is probably a misnomer as the tumor arises primarily from the inner wall of blood vessels. In the classic or traditional form of this disease, the tumor arises primarily on the lower legs of elderly males and follows a relatively limited and painless course. Tumors are treated easily with local radiation to the involved areas or, if more extensive, by chemotherapy with drugs such as vinblastine (Valban). The tumor is easily controlled, with most individuals dying of diseases other than Kaposi's sarcoma.

Endemic African. A second form of Kaposi's sarcoma occurs commonly in equatorial Africa and comprises up to 10 percent of all cancers among the Bantu tribes of Zaire and Uganda. The disease occurs in younger individuals and generally follows a more rapidly growing course in African patients. The geographical distribution of cases in Africa parallels the so-called "lymphoma belt" of Burkitt's lymphoma, a tumor which is closely associated with Epstein-Barr virus. It has therefore been postulated that Kaposi's sarcoma may also be associated with a virus.

Epidemic. Recently a similarly aggressive form of Kaposi's sarcoma has been seen among homosexually active males in association with the acquired immunodeficiency syndrome. The tumor ordinarily does not occur in this age range (under the age of sixty) in any substantial number and can, therefore, be called a true epidemic. In AIDS the tumor, which looks very similar to the classic form of Kaposi's sarcoma, may occur anywhere on the body and frequently involves internal organs at a fairly early stage in its development. Microscopically, the tumor appears identical to that seen among older Jewish men or African patients. However, the characteristics of the tumor are such that many experts feel that it may, in fact, be different.

Description

The appearance and progression of Kaposi's sarcoma are largely determined by the situation in which the tumor arises. In the classical form occurring in elderly Caucasian males, the tumor grows slowly and is generally restricted to the lower legs. The endemic African form of Kaposi's sarcoma has more widespread skin involvement and may start with lymph node swelling.

The epidemic form of Kaposi's sarcoma associated with AIDS usually appears as painless purple to brownish, slightly raised spots on the skin or mucous membranes of the mouth. The skin lesions may appear anywhere on the body including the skin of the feet, legs or arms, face, neck, chest,or back. Lymph nodes and internal organs can also be involved. In most cases they do not cause the patient any discomfort. The gastrointestinal tract is the most common site of internal involvement with Kaposi's sarcoma, and oftentimes it can be detected only through direct examination with a specialized instrument called an endoscope. On rare occasions the lungs and other organs are involved, but usually this does not occur until the disease has spread in its final stages. Individuals who develop new or unusual appearing discolorations of bumps on their skin (and belong to any one of the high-risk groups for AIDS) should consult their physician or dermatologist for a skin biopsy to rule out the possibility of Kaposi's sarcoma. This is particularly important as these lesions generally do not cause any symptoms.

The course of the tumor varies from individual to individual. However, among homosexual men Kaposi's sarcoma tends to spread more rapidly than among the elderly Jewish population. Because of this, it is recommended that patients with the diagnosis of Kaposi's sarcoma be evaluated for underlying immune abnormalities associated with AIDS and, if detected, should be referred to a practicing oncologist (cancer specialist) or university teaching center for appropriate treatment.

Why Does It Occur?

The cause of Kaposi's sarcoma is, as yet, not clearly defined. There is mounting evidence that underlying immunodeficiency may allow the development of Kaposi's sarcoma as well as other cancers. Cases of Kaposi's sarcoma have occurred in people receiving immunosuppressive drugs to prevent rejection of a transplanted kidney and among those receiving cancer chemotherapy, which also suppresses the immune system. The geographical distribution of Kaposi's sarcoma may be related to viral infections. There is some evidence that cytomegalovirus, a common virus which ordinarily does not cause a problem in the healthy host, may cause cells to become malignant (cancerous), as in Kaposi's sarcoma when immunodeficiency is present. It is believed that repeated exposure to this virus or other similar viruses (such as through the secretions of homosexual men) may contribute to the immunodeficiency and possibly the malignancies associated with AIDS. In addition, there may be a certain genetic predisposition to develop Kaposi's sarcoma in individuals with

AIDS. A disproportionate prevalence of one tissue typing antigen, HAL-DR5, has been reported among patients with AIDS who develop Kaposi's sarcoma. Further investigations in the epidemiology, virology, and immunology of patients with AIDS and Kaposi's sarcoma may ultimately yield answers as to why this unusual tumor occurs in the AIDS setting.

III. CENTRAL NERVOUS SYSTEM HIV INFECTION

AIDS patients are also affected by a central nervous system (CNS) infection of the AIDS virus. In the early days of the disease, many people with AIDS exhibited signs of depression, complicated sometimes by memory loss and a sense of despondency and listlessness. Physicians attributed these symptoms to patients trying to cope with the news that they had a terminal disease. As researchers discovered more and more about the viral cause of AIDS, they found that HIV can infect the brain and the central nervous system. HIV is now known to seek out and attack nerve cells, causing dementia, which can range from mild to severe.

Although people with AIDS still have a very a natural response to their diagnosis with feelings of depression and disorientation, physicians and therapists are now alert to the possibility that at some point these symptoms may also reflect the effect of the virus infecting the central nervous system.

Researchers now seek treatments that will not only block the effects of the virus on cells of the immune system, but will also cross what is called the "blood-brain barrier" to stop the action of HIV in the brain and central nervous system. One of the current drugs being tested, AZT, has been found to cross that barrier.

[Editor's note: AZT has recently been approved by the FDA for limited use for some AIDS patients].

Coping with ARC

Buck Nunes and Chuck Frutchey

What Is ARC?

ARC is AIDS-related complex; it describes a variety of conditions resulting from infection with the AIDS virus. These conditions are different and usually less severe than the specific diseases present with AIDS. At the present time, ARC has no "official" definition. Simply stated, ARC is usually a less severe reaction to the AIDS virus and is a sexually transmitted disease that can also be spread by sharing needles. This makes ARC a very broad catch-all category that includes people with a wide range of symptoms.

What Are the Symptoms of ARC?

Many symptoms of ARC are the same as those for AIDS. They include:

- unexplained, persistent fatigue;

- unexplained fever, shaking chills, or drenching night sweats lasting longer than several weeks;

Excerted from the booklet, "Coping with ARC," published by the San Francisco AIDS Foundation. Reprinted with permission.

- unexplained weight loss greater than ten pounds in less than one or two months;

- swollen glands (enlarged lymph nodes usually in the neck, armpits, or groin) which are otherwise unexplained and last more than two weeks;

- persistent white spots or unusual blemishes in the mouth;

- persistent diarrhea for no known reason;

- unusual bruising or bleeding.

Remember, these symptoms are common in other illnesses as well. In AIDS or ARC, however, they tend to be longer lasting, more severe, or recurrent. Any disease symptoms should be evaluated by a qualified doctor.

What happens to people with ARC? There is no clear and consistent way that ARC progresses. The illness differs from person to person. Some people have only a mild or occasional condition while others become quite sick (and disabled). From 10 to 20 percent of people with ARC have developed AIDS within two years of initial diagnosis. [Editor's note: Based on further study, researchers now believe that the percentage of people with ARC who progress to full-blown AIDS is somewhat higher]. Other people have not worsened. At this time the long-term prospects for ARC are not known.

What Health Problems Might Be Expected?

How someone with ARC feels may fluctuate from day to day. Some people may be ill enough, at least part of the time, to qualify for disability; for others, symptoms are minor and do not prevent them from continuing with their normal activities. Some infections might occur from time to time, but many of these can be treated with existing medications.

Are There Specific Diseases Associated with ARC?

Several diseases are associated with ARC, and their presence may indicate some immune depression. They include:

Persistent Generalized Lymphadenopathy (swollen lymph nodes). Any time an infection occurs, some lymph nodes swell up, usually the ones nearest the infection (lymph nodes are located in many areas of the body). After a bad infection, these nodes may stay swollen for several weeks. Persistent lymphadenopathy is usually defined as lymph nodes that are chronically swollen for more than six months in at least two locations, not including the groin. The lymph nodes may be sore or visible externally, but this is not always true.

Thrush. This is a yeast infection in the mouth caused by an organism called candida albicans. [Editor's note: The presence of thrush alone does not always indicate ARC or AIDS; thrush is common in babies, diabetics, and people who have received high doses of antibiotics.] Candida is a normal fungus in the body, usually residing in the gut with many other organisms. During periods of lowered immunity, candida sometimes flourishes in other parts of the body. It can cause vaginitis (vaginal yeast infection), "jock itch," or sinus infections. (Sometimes candida infections occur soon after taking antibiotics, which kill the bacteria that control candida.) When it is on the tongue or gums, it is called thrush. It looks like a gray or white patchy coating that cannot be scraped off. It might only cover a part of the tongue, or the entire inside of the mouth. This same infection, if it progresses to the throat or the lungs, can qualify for a diagnosis of AIDS.

Hairy Leukoplakia. Sometimes mistaken for thrush, hairy leukoplakia is a white patch that appears on the sides of the tongue. It is usually thicker than thrush and also cannot be scraped off. It is called "hairy" because of its appearance, which is like wet cotton or velvet. In some people, hairy leukoplakia may disappear after awhile. It is caused by a combination of two viruses living together. This condition is a strong indicator of an AIDS viral infection, and it is not known if it is contagious.

Shingles. Shingles is caused by the same virus that causes chicken pox: herpes zoster. After a bout of chicken pox, usually at an early age, the virus retreats into the nervous system where it lies dormant. It can re-emerge during periods of high stress or depressed immunity. Shingles is a disease seen more often in older people whose immune systems are declining. It has recently been seen in many young and middle-aged people who are at increased risk for AIDS. The disease causes painful herpes-like lesions, most commonly around the torso, following the lines of the nerves, but can occur elsewhere on the body as well.

Idiopathic Thrombocytopenic Purpura (ITP). ITP is a condition in which the body produces antibodies against its own platelets, which are the blood cells that cause blood clotting. The primary symptom is easy bruising, although blood in stools, bleeding gums, or slow healing of wounds can also be symptoms. ITP can be caused by many things, and is not necessarily AIDS-related.

While it is generally uncommon in adult men, ITP has been seen more and more in adult men who are at an increased risk for AIDS. It sometimes resolves on its own.

These illnesses can occur and be unrelated to infection with the AIDS virus, so it is important that an AIDS-aware and knowledgeable doctor determine if the illness is actually AIDS-related. [Editor's note: Patients can receive the best care from their doctors when they are open and honest, informing their physicians about their personal history and concerns, including sexual and drug use history].

How Is ARC Diagnosed?

Because the symptoms of ARC and AIDS are similar to those of so many other illnesses, a diagnosis is difficult to make. With AIDS there are specific diseases whose presence is used to make an AIDS diagnosis. By definition, people with ARC do not have Kaposi's sarcoma (KS), pneumocystis carinii pneumonia (PCP), toxoplasmosis, or lymphoma. If your diagnosis included these illnesses, you would be classified as having AIDS.

With ARC the situation is not so clear. A diagnosis of ARC, therefore, is often based on the opinion of the physician. This is why it is important to see an AIDS-knowledgeable physician if any of the suspicious symptoms or diseases are present. Depending on an individual's specific situation, the doctor may wish to run various tests to evaluate the condition and clarify the diagnosis. At this time, there is no simple test for ARC or AIDS, and a diagnosis is based on many pieces of information, including personal history, medical symptoms, and laboratory tests. Doctors and researchers are now trying to agree on a standard definition of ARC to make this process easier.

Are There Any Treatments for ARC?

Many of the illnesses and conditions that people with ARC may get are treatable with common medications. However, there is still no effective treatment for the underlying immune depression.

Several experimental drugs and protocols are being tested in the hopes that one or more of them may be useful. If you are interested in being involved in an experimental testing program, you should first discuss the possibility with your doctor. Experimental treatment programs are offered at only a few locations and to a limited number of people. Each participant must meet certain criteria to be included. An individual's doctor can usually offer advice on eligibility.

Some people have chosen to go to another area or a foreign country to obtain drugs or treatments that are not available in their location. Again, private physicians should be consulted before such decisions are made.

What About Alternative Therapies?

Some people decide to pursue alternative therapies for treating ARC. These might include acupuncture, vitamins, visualization, or other approaches. Presently, little is known about the effectiveness of alternative treatments.

There are several issues that individuals should be aware of if they decide to pursue alternative treatments. Most of these treatments have not been rigorously tested under controlled conditions, and it is unlikely that this will happen in the near future. Therefore, it is important that individuals research any alternative treatment that they might be considering. (This is also good advice for medical treatments.) Alternative practitioners can be consulted about any questions or concerns about the treatment. It is also important, whenever more than one person is providing treatments, that they consult with one another about the condition of the patient. This will help avoid situations such as an herbalist giving an herb that will counteract the medicine a doctor prescribes, or vice-versa.

Is Medical Supervision Needed by People with ARC?

Yes. First of all, individuals will need to see a doctor to know if they have ARC. It is not a diagnosis someone can make on his or her own. Furthermore, various problems may occur from time to time and require a doctor's attention. Even individuals who are seeing alternative practitioners will need a doctor to run tests to evaluate their clinical condition. It is of great benefit to continue to see one doctor who has followed the course of an individual's disease. Many doctors will work closely with alternative practitioners.

How Can People with ARC Take Care of Their Health?

There are a number of things that constitute good health habits. These include adequate rest and sleep, plenty of exercise (to the extent of ability), and good nutrition. All of these have an effect on the immune system.

Stress is also an important factor. Excessive or prolonged stress can depress the immune system's ability to respond. The stress of everyday living, a disease diagnosis, as well as physical stress, can all contribute to this problem.

There are techniques for reducing and managing stress as well as avoiding stressful situations. Groups and organizations are available to provide training in these techniques.

It is also important for individuals to keep from reinfecting themselves with the AIDS virus (through unprotected sexual activities or shared-needle IV-drug use) because it is possible that reinfection may worsen the ARC.

What About Drugs and Alcohol?

Alcohol, most street drugs, and some medicines have an adverse effect on the immune system. At a time when health should be maintained as much as possible, it is advisable for individuals to avoid or minimize use of these substances. If someone is having trouble controlling drug or alcohol use, there are agencies that can help. If someone does take the risk of using drugs intravenously, needles should not be shared. Needle-sharing is a direct route for the transmission of the AIDS virus. Drugs and alcohol can also affect judgment concerning good health practices and safe sexual activity.

Should I Take the Antibody Test?

The AIDS antibody test shows whether someone has been infected by the AIDS virus. This test, if used in combination with other medical tests and observations, can sometimes be useful in determining whether or not a person has ARC. Often a physician will recommend the test for this reason. This test cannot determine whether or not someone will go on to develop AIDS, but people who test positive are warned that they are probably infectious, and that they need to take appropriate precautions to prevent transmitting the virus.

Because of the possibility of discrimination or loss of insurance, an individual should obtain definite assurance that confidentiality can be protected before taking the test. (Many health departments throughout the country provide the antibody test with guaranteed anonymity.) A negative test result is no guarantee that the AIDS virus is not present since it may take several months for antibodies to develop. Those individuals who receive a negative test result but have other signs of ARC should discuss the situation with their doctors. It may be advisable to take the test again a few months later. [Editor's note: Individuals who are at high risk for AIDS, have signs of ARC, and receive a negative test result, should still consider themselves to be possibly infectious. They should continue to avoid all activities that might expose themselves or others to the AIDS virus].

What Might Be the Sources of Stress in Everyday Life?

Most people experience stress as a result of an ARC diagnosis. This stress may be caused by a number of factors; it may range from mild to severe and can include both mental and physical stress. There is the fear of the condition developing into full-blown AIDS. The everyday stress of being sick is probably the most immediate and continuing kind of stress to be experienced. Depending on the severity of the illness, there may be days that are worse than others. Some people may have trouble getting out of bed. At other times they may feel as if there is nothing wrong. These reactions may be directly caused by the physical symptoms of the illness, such as weight loss and fever.

However, depression, anxiety, and other psychological reactions to being ill can produce the same results. It may not always be easy to tell the difference, but it is important that both patients and their doctors be aware that both conditions might occur.

Because ARC is so loosely defined, many people experience great anxiety over not knowing exactly how to evaluate their medical conditions. Likewise, their doctors may be unclear about how to interpret symptoms or test results. While this uncertainty may be a significant source of stress, it can also be a motivator to increase awareness of a condition and the ways to deal with it.

The reaction received from other people about an ARC diagnosis may take many different forms. Some people, possibly including close family and friends, may exhibit fear and avoidance. This in turn can affect the diagnosed person's self-esteem, leading to questions about self-worth. It is important to remember that not everyone will feel this way about you. Other friends will continue to be loving and supportive. You may also find it helpful to meet other people with ARC and share experiences with them.

Another common source of stress can be the extensive questioning and testing that occurs during diagnosis and treatment. Often the patients feel that health professionals are prying into their lives; they may get tired of being stuck with so many needles and being asked to endure so many tests. While it is important for patients to voice their frustrations and not let them remain bottled up, especially when doctors and other staff are not sensitive to particular needs, it is equally important to realize that everyone has the same goal in mind: improved health of the patient.

How Can I Deal with Stress?

The stress that may result from having ARC will not be the first stress a person has experienced in life. Some people cope with stress better than others. Many people have situations from the past they can draw on that have taught them how to constructively cope with stress. The details may be different, but the coping methods are the same.

It is important to remember that there is always more than one choice to be made. For every situation that causes stress, there will be steps you can take to counteract that stress. Like other aspects of your life, you can have control over your reaction to stressful events and situations in your life.

An easy and effective method for dealing with stress is talking. Verbalizing fears, anxieties, and frustrations has a way of bringing them into focus and clarifying them. Talking with a professional counselor, a friend, or a group of people are all effective ways to decrease stress. There are also established techniques, such as relaxation exercises, guided visualization, and massage, that are helpful in controlling stress and depression. Many people have found these techniques to be an important part of their ability to cope with ARC. Several individuals and organizations offer training in how to use these methods. By learning what triggers stress for them, individuals can learn how to cope better with stressful situations.

Confusion is often an initial reaction to diagnosis. The combined effects of discovering they are ill, an uncertain future, and no clear treatment plan can make it difficult for people with ARC to develop a clear picture of their situation. With the help of personal doctors and others, they can develop a clearer picture of what ARC is and how it will affect their lives. It is important for people to overcome this initial confusion so that they will be better able to make important decisions about their treatment and future plans. Some people will react to having ARC by trying to diminish its importance or by pretending that it doesn't exist at all. This is known as denial. It can be even more debilitating than confusion because a person in denial may refuse to consider appropriate plans or suggestions. For anyone who is initially frightened by the diagnosis (which is common), denial may seem like an attractive route to follow. While denial may be a reasonable or understandable reaction, people with ARC should remember that it may prevent them from making important health decisions, such as what treatment to get. It is important to be alert to the possibility that denial might exist.

In dealing with stress, rest, exercise, and proper nutrition can be very helpful. Staying busy and exercising are time-honored remedies for everyday stress and depression. Strenuous exercise for a short period of time each day has a positive effect on the immune system. Proper nutrition also has a powerful effect on the way someone feels, both physically and mentally. Doctors and nutritionists can offer advice about the quality of current diets.

Who Should Be Told About My Illness?

One issue that needs to be faced is who to tell about the diagnosis. Different factors will be involved depending on the persons being told. Some people will decide to be very open about having ARC while others will decide they only want a few people to know. Whether or not to tell friends or family may depend on how close the relationship is. Close friends or family members may be told first, and others later at times that seem appropriate. Important considerations are the amount of trust involved in the relationship, the level of the relationship, a person's openness about sexual lifestyle and possible drug use, and the potential risk of informing people of the diagnosis. Some people with ARC do not care to keep their diagnosis confidential at all.

As with any disease that may be contagious, dentists and other health-care providers should be told of an ARC diagnosis. In the course of their duties, these people may be intimately exposed to possibly infectious secretions, such as blood, and can take precautions if they know the patient has a contagious disease.

Whether or not employers or co-workers are told may require more thought. Depending on the state of an individual's health, there may be no need for them to know. However, a person's anxiety may be reduced if they are under no pressure to keep a secret. In fact, your co-workers and employer may be a potential source of support. Most people with ARC want, need, and are able to work. Some are fortunate enough to work out schedules tailored to their needs.

Others may face discrimination by employers and co-workers. There are legal remedies available to combat this discrimination. Many communities ban discrimination on the basis of medical condition or disability. Some communities prohibit discrimination on the basis of sexual orientation or even a specific AIDS diagnosis. When an individual suspects discrimination, representatives of local AIDS service organizations, fair housing and employment offices, and city attorneys may be helpful.

What Is the Likelihood of Developing AIDS?

Many people with ARC worry about developing full-blown AIDS. The best information available suggests that 10 to 20 percent of people with ARC will go on to get AIDS within two years of diagnosis. [Editor's note: Some recent studies indicate that this percentage may be higher]. The long-term prospects of having ARC are not known, but dwelling on the likelihood of developing AIDS will only increase anxiety. Concentrating instead on maintaining or improving health, reducing stress, practicing safe sex, and developing a positive attitude, may help reduce fears about the future.

Will I Be Able to Continue Working?

For most people, having ARC will not interfere with their being able to work or keep a job. The majority of people with ARC do not experience significant fatigue or other debilitating symptoms. For others, steady work will be difficult or impossible. They may experience such profound fatigue that just getting out of bed can be a chore. Some people with ARC may find themselves at neither of these extremes, but somewhere in between. Another factor is that individuals' energy levels may change from day to day.

If someone with ARC is presently working and having no difficulty, there is probably no reason to stop working or cutting back. If the condition worsens, however, it may be wise to make arrangements to work fewer hours or to change jobs. People with ARC should be advised not to push themselves too hard or they may risk making themselves sicker. Some people who are unable to work regularly find that they need to do something to keep from getting bored; this might include volunteer work or other activities.

Without Work, How Can People with ARC Support Themselves?

Most people do not have the financial resources to get by without a steady job. For those who are unable to work, resources exist for financial assistance as well as agencies that can help in applying for such assistance. Unlike a diagnosis of AIDS, an ARC diagnosis does not automatically qualify someone for government disability payments. Most people who are disabled with ARC are eligible for these programs. However, eligibility may take longer to demonstrate with an ARC diagnosis. (See Section Seven, A PRACTICAL PERSPECTIVE.)

Can Someone with ARC Still Have Sex?

A diagnosis of ARC does not mean that someone's sex life must end. Some people, out of fear or misinformation, think that their only option is to become celibate. Although they may be contagious, there are many ways to have sex that do not transmit the AIDS virus. The safe-sex guidelines developed by medical experts enable anyone to have sex without fear of infection. (See Section Five, "Safe-Sex Guidelines.") It is important to *always* practice safe sex; otherwise, reinfection might occur and make ARC conditions worse. Unsafe sex could also infect someone else. Because of a compromised immune system, people with ARC or AIDS are more at risk of catching diseases in an unsafe sexual contact than a healthy person.

Telling a potential sex partner about an ARC diagnosis may seem, at first, frightening or difficult, but it is important to do so for the sake of the other person involved. Whether you tell your partner or not, however, you should always have safe sex.

What About Support?

The burden of dealing with a chronic health problem should be shared with others. Friends and family may want to help. Often, they are afraid of overstepping some unstated boundary. People with ARC can make it easier for themselves and for their friends and family by giving them permission to provide support when it is needed. They may also need suggestions about what they can do. Support can come from many places.

Lover/Spouse. Partners may have many of the same emotional needs that their diagnosed lover has. Individuals should not be afraid to support each other. They should consider getting help from others so that problems do not overwhelm their relationship.

Roommates. It is important to discuss with roommates all aspects of the disease, emotional needs, physical needs and limitations, and fear of contagion. Understanding each other's needs and fears can help maintain a good relationship and avoid breakdown in communications.

Family/Relatives. How and when to tell family members about a diagnosis of ARC will depend on the existing relationship with them. It is okay not to tell them immediately; the diagnosed person can be the judge of the best time. Knowing how someone else has told his parents may be helpful in making the decision. Family members may have limited ideas concerning what should be done and about how to help. Information referrals and other resources are available to answer their questions and help them to understand the situation.

Extended Family. These are the people who help someone get through life's problems; now is no different. If they are informed of the diagnosis, it is helpful to tell them just how they can be supportive. They should be told that it is okay to respond the way they always have. Given the opportunity, they may offer nurturing, love, and affection in positive ways.

Support Groups. Interacting with others in support groups can provide a perspective, help ease fear and uncertainty, and reduce isolation with the disease. They can provide an environment for learning the experiences of others in similar situations and getting a type of support sometimes not available from one's own friends and family. Many organizations also offer one-on-one counseling. Other organizations offer emotional support for families and other concerned loved ones.

Others with ARC. Many people with ARC find great support and comfort in developing personal friendships with other people with ARC. This gives them the opportunity to share and examine similar experiences, feelings, and problems. Having the same diagnosis seems to develop common bonds and a level of understanding that is unique.

Individual Counseling. Seeing a counselor or therapist on a regular basis can provide a safe and secure environment to discuss problems and anxieties. For some people a professional rather than a personal relationship makes it easier to discuss sensitive issues.

Summary

Although ARC describes a wide range of illnesses, from mild to severe, everyone who is diagnosed with ARC needs to remember that it is a serious condition. Many people with ARC have only a mild illness and are able to work and continue with normal daily activities. For others, however, a diagnosis of ARC means medical problems and financial hardship. For the person with ARC, the more that is known about the illness, the better one is equipped to make decisions about health.

The medical aspects of ARC are not the only factors to be aware of. Psychological well-being and overall attitude will determine how well someone with ARC will be. Changes in health may come from day to day or month to month. In addition, research is constantly changing what we know about ARC and our ability to treat it.

Medical Impact of AIDS on Hemophilia

Shelby L. Dietrich, M.D.

Hemophilia is the medical term used to describe a group of disorders that affect people from birth and disrupt blood clotting or coagulation. The disorders make a person likely to experience bleeding that does not stop without special treatments.

The major bleeding disorders include hemophilia A or classic hemophilia, hemophilia B, and von Willebrand's disease. Each results from a lack of proteins in the body. Hemophilia A is a deficiency or lack of factor VIII, a protein normally present in the blood. This blood factor is necessary for normal clotting mechanisms to operate. By comparison, hemophilia B represents a deficiency in factor IX, another protein also essential for normal clotting. Both these disorders are transmitted as female sex-linked conditions, meaning that the disease can be passed from mothers to sons. In addition, a mother's daughters can be carriers of the disorders (as carriers, women are not affected by the disease themselves, but are able to pass it to others). As a result, hemophilia A and B are found in males only.

By contrast, von Willebrand's disease is a combined disorder of factor VIII deficiency and the improper functioning of the platelets (small disks in the blood that help clotting). This disease occurs in both males and females, and is transmitted through genes at birth. These three disorders comprise 95 percent of the diagnosed cases of clotting disorders that occur at birth.

Clinically, the disorder appears with a spectrum of laboratory and clinical findings ranging from mild to severe. Within a given family the deficiency is similar in all affected males. Carrier females sometimes have levels of factor VIII or factor IX low enough to cause problems with bleeding. In severe cases the disorder is usually diagnosed either at birth because of family history or during the first year of life.

Treatment

Replacement of the missing factor corrects the abnormal clotting mechanism; therefore, treatment of hemophilia consists of intravenous (IV) use of the clotting factor. Effective treatment became possible about two decades ago when cryoprecipitate, a blood component, and plasma clotting concentrates of factors VIII and IX were developed.

With the availability of these materials, the hemophiliac could for the first time lead a normal life, could undergo reconstructive orthopedic surgery to achieve a near-normal life span. Home treatment became a reality, and most severe hemophilia A and B patients were able to have IV-injections at home, school, or at work, given by parents or the patients themselves. Home or supervised self-treatment freed hemophiliacs from their dependence on the hospital for treatment and opened new horizons of active lifestyles.

Powerful therapeutic agents, such as clotting factor concentrates and blood components, are not without risks and side effects. Cryoprecipitate and fresh frozen plasma are useful in the treatment of von Willebrand's disease and mild forms of factor IX deficiency. Both these components are prepared by blood banks from single-donor blood donations. Single-donor products are less likely to transmit certain donor infections, such as hepatitis, to infrequent recipients than are multiple-donor products, such as those concentrates made from pooled plasma (combinations of blood donations from several people). But neither of these components can be heat-treated, and people often have allergic reactions to blood components.

Factors VIII and IX concentrates are prepared by drug companies from plasma pooled from thousands of donors. Each lot is distributed into many vials, submitted to a freeze-drying process, and analyzed for its different components. Concentrates are stable at room temperatures, easy to make whole again, cause only rare allergic reactions, and make self-injection programs convenient. The disadvantages of the concentrates relate mostly to the large donor pool, since a single dose of concentrate is more likely than cryoprecipitate to contain viruses of hepatitis B, or non-A non-B hepatitis, and—prior to the heat treatment of the concentrates—the AIDS virus.

Heat treatment of factors VIII and IX concentrates, since 1982 for hemophiliacs, was primarily begun to lower the risk of non-A non-B hepatitis, but coincidentally was found to be effective against the AIDS virus. Unfortunately, heat treatment was found to offer no protection against the primary target, non-A non-B hepatitis. All blood and plasma in the United States is now screened (and has been since 1985) for presence of antibodies to HIV, the AIDS virus.

Effects of AIDS on Hemophiliacs

Before AIDS appeared in the hemophilia population, the average adult hemophiliac led a fairly normal life, controlling bleeding problems with self-injection of factor VIII or factor IX concentrate and not being overly concerned with the problems of hepatitis. The younger patients, born after concentrates became available, are growing up without significant orthopedic disability, enjoying a normal school and childhood experience.

With the first appearance of AIDS in the hemophilia population in 1982, it was soon clear that AIDS was a major threat to the well-being of people exposed to blood products. Currently, it is estimated that 75 to 80 percent of the heavily-treated factor VIII patients in the United States are seropositive to the AIDS virus, meaning that they have been exposed to it and are probably infectious. Statistics change daily as to the number of cases of AIDS in hemophiliacs, according to the Centers for Disease Control. The majority of hemophilia AIDS-related cases have been diagnosed in patients lacking factor VIII, although a few AIDS cases have occurred among patients with factor IX deficiency and those with von Willebrand's disease.

Studies of the history of seroconversion to the AIDS virus (showing exposure to it) indicate that hemophiliacs began to be exposed to the virus in 1979 and then many more became exposed rapidly in the years 1981 and 1982. The natural history of AIDS viral infection in hemophiliacs is still unknown, leaving heavily-treated hemophiliacs in a position of agonizing uncertainty over their future health.

Sexual transmission of the AIDS virus to spouses of hemophiliacs has been documented, but it appears to be an infrequent occurrence. There have been no documented cases of household transmission of the AIDS virus.

Recommendations for Persons with Hemophilia

The best and most sound medical advice at this time appears to be that someone with hemophilia should continue appropriate treatment of bleeding problems, should observe safe sexual practices, and should keep in close contact with his physician or treatment center. Spouses are advised to defer pregnancy until further information is available.

Section Four

Treatment:
A Therapeutic
Perspective

The single most important thing the family can offer is their willingness to go through this experience with their loved one... Treating the patient as if you expect him or her to live is essential. The family need not believe the patient will recover; they need only believe that he or she can recover... You are part of the patient's support system, so it is important that you support health and recovery.

"Alternative Therapies: Another Approach"

Treatment and Prevention of AIDS
Medical Treatment of Kaposi's Sarcoma
Choosing Alternative Therapies

Treatment and Prevention of AIDS

John Ziegler, M.D.

Treatment strategies for patients with AIDS and AIDS-related complex (ARC) are aimed at three broad targets: prevention of infection by the AIDS retrovirus; prevention of damage to the immune system following viral infection; and treatment of complicating illnesses such as opportunistic infections and cancer.

At the present time, the most important and most successful approach is to prevent infection in the first place. We know that the AIDS retrovirus is spread in two ways: by blood or blood products from infected individuals and by sexual transmission.

In the United States the epidemic has remained confined largely to indivuals in certain risk groups who may be exposed to the virus through sexual intimacy and/or contact with contaminated blood or blood products. The latter include blood transfusion recipients, infants of infected mothers, hemophiliacs, and IV-drug users who share contaminated needles. In this country sexual transmission is most common among gay and bisexual men (particularly those who have had many partners and who have exchanged semen during anal intercourse). Heterosexual transmission is not common in the

This article first appeared in *FOCUS: A Review of AIDS Research*, March 1986, Volume 1, Number 4.

United States as yet, although statistics are changing to encompass the hetero-sexual population as well. Heterosexual transmission seems to occur mostly in female partners of infected males, but it can be transmitted in either direction. There is no evidence of *casual* spread of the virus either within or outside of these risk groups.

The development of a test to detect persons who have antibodies to the AIDS retrovirus (and therefore are presumed to be infectious) has permitted screening of blood donors. This measure has effectively protected the blood supply. Blood products are now also heat-treated, a process which inactivates the virus and makes use of them safe. This means that new cases of transfusion-related cases or among hemophiliacs should be rare or absent. Cases that will be seen in the next four to five years will be those exposed or infected prior to the screening of the blood supply in 1985. [Editor's note: Current research suggests an incubation period of up to ten years; therefore, symptoms could manifest as late as 1995.]

The prevention of exposure to the virus in other risk groups through education and behavior changes has been more difficult. Public health measures, such as closing bath houses to discourage high-risk sexual activities and supplying sterile needles to intravenous drug addicts, prompt social and political controversy. Educational measures, such as pamphlets, media messages, and counseling, have made some headway, particularly in discouraging unsafe sexual activity. Ongoing studies in several American cities have documented substantial changes in reported sexual behavior from high-risk to low-risk activities.

There remains, however, a great deal more to be accomplished in the area of primary prevention. In San Francisco the prevalence of AIDS antibodies among an estimated 10,000 intravenous drug addicts is about 10 percent. In New York and New Jersey, the rate is 50 percent. The Department of Public Health has undertaken programs to prevent further spread of the virus in this group.

The next most obvious preventive measure is a vaccine. The phenomenal progress in the field of molecular biology in the last decade has permitted the cloning (obtaining a group of identical items from a single original) and sequencing of the AIDS retrovirus; thus we know its molecular anatomy, or structure, in some detail. The most vulnerable portion of the virus, its outer "envelope" protein, seems to vary considerably in different isolates of the virus. Scientists are now searching to find a "constant" portion of the viral envelope that could be used as a vaccine. The development and testing of vaccines take many years (at least ten years in the case of hepatitis vaccine). Thus, while there is promise of success, many more individuals will be at risk of infection before a safe and effective vaccine will be ready.

The next strategy in the treatment hierarchy is to halt progression from asymptomatic (with no disease symptoms) infection with the AIDS virus to actual illness with disease symptoms. We know that the virus attacks primarily the helper T-lymphocyte, a cell which acts as the director of many immune responses. The incubation period from infection to illness varies from several months to more than six years, and possibly up to ten years. In the test tube, the AIDS virus will kill its host cell, although some cells may escape and enter a state of "latent" infection in which the virus remains but does not actively reproduce. The virus can then be reactivated in these cells by various stimuli.

Although we do not understand what happens in the body, we can infer that the chain of events is similar to what happens in test tubes: infected T-cells producing virus (estimated to be about one in a thousand cells) are killed. Cells containing latent virus may become reactivated with time, so that duplicating virus can infect other T-cells. The net result is a slow but relentless destruction of the entire helper T-cell population. Researchers presume that other infections or stimuli that disturb the immune system can act as "cofactors" (agents or events that assist the primary infection) and aggravate the latent state by periodically reactivating virus production.

There are a number of other theories that may explain the progressive immune destruction in AIDS. These include an "autoimmune" attack by the immune system itself against the infected helper T-cells; alterations of the immune response by viral products released into the circulation; and direct disruption of immune function by the virus.

Given the current limitations to our knowledge, it is safe to say that the ultimate cause and course of the immune system dysfunction is unknown. Therefore, it is difficult to devise specific therapies to avert immune impairment.

Antiviral Therapy

One potentially promising approach is to block viral reproduction with antiviral drugs or with specific antibodies. There are compounds that inhibit the activity of the viral enzyme, "reverse transcriptase," that is essential for reproduction.

Another drug may attack the "proviral" stage when the genetic material of the virus is integrated into host cell DNA. Other agents apparently attack the virus physically, and alter its envelope coating.

All of these drugs were discovered in the laboratory, and their effectiveness and toxicity in man are unknown. At the same time, many laboratories seek neutralizing antibodies that attach to the virus and prevent its infectivity. The entire area of antiviral therapy is now in its earliest stages of clinical trial. It is critically important to learn how the body handles these drugs, whether they exert an antiviral effect, what the best dosage is for optimal effect, and, more importantly, the toxic side effects of the agents. It is important that the same scientific rigor be applied to clinical studies (with human subjects) as it is in laboratory research (just using test tubes).

To reach valid results about data, investigators must select a representative sample from the population, monitor the effects of any intervention, and interpret their results in relation to a comparable control sample.

To fulfill this last objective, trials must often include a control group to ensure that the experimental drug really achieves the desired effect. This group may receive treatment with a standard agent, or with a "placebo" or dummy pill. Usually, neither the investigator nor the patients will know what treatment they are receiving. Assignment of patients for treatment with the experimental drug or placebo must be made by random methods, since investigators would introduce a bias by selecting patients themselves.

While these methods may seem cumbersome to the non-researcher, the inferences made from the trial must be sufficiently convincing to bring about a change in treatment practices. A patient who agrees to enter a trial must know that the treatments offered are either "state-of-the-art" or an experimental treatment whose effect and toxicity are unknown. As a trial participant, each subject becomes a courageous partner with the researcher in the scientific pursuit of better therapy.

Immunomodulators

Early in the epidemic researchers recognized a progressive imbalance in the T-lymphocyte populations and a wide array of immunologic dysfunctions. Many researchers felt that stimulation of the faltering immune system by various agents known to boost immune reactions might be therapeutic. A large number of such immunomodulators were tested in the clinic, but there were no consistent benefits in any patient.

We now know that this approach must be re-examined. The immune system does not operate in an on-off mode but is in a state of dynamic balance. When disturbed by any foreign stimulus, a swift response, involving several different cooperating cells, is set in motion. With AIDS these cells are deficient and non-responsive, behaving as though they were disoriented and preoccupied. The exact mechanism by which this state of immune dysfunction occurs has been elusive, but all evidence implicates the helper T-cells and another set of cells known as macrophages. In particular, the helper T-cells fail to recognize antigens, or foreign substances, and fail to make an important hormone called interleukin-2 (IL-2). This hormone acts as a signal to other T-cells to respond to the antigen. However, clinical trials of IL-2 have been disappointing. Much more must be known about the cause and course of the immune deficiency in AIDS before other treatments with immune stimulators are tried.

Treatment of Illnesses

The final strategy is to treat the many illnesses that result from immune deficiency. The most dangerous of these are the opportunistic infections by microbes that do not cause disease in persons with normally functioning immune systems. Successful treatment for opportunistic infections requires cooperation between antibiotics and host defenses. In an individual with a damaged immune system, treatment must be prolonged and intensive; in AIDS patients many of these treatments often have significant side effects.

Despite these obstacles, a number of clinical trials have succeeded in slowing infections and producing clinical improvement. Unfortunately, relapse and simultaneous infection with several microbes are common. Thus the prognosis for patients with opportunistic infections is poor. Present trials attempt to identify individuals at high risk and to treat them "prophylactically" or preventively with suppressive antibiotics to prevent infection.

Patients with AIDS, and particularly gay men, are also plagued by two types of cancer: Kaposi's sarcoma and Hodgkin's lymphoma, a cancer of the lymph system. These neoplasms (cancers) prey upon persons with damaged immune systems. Unfortunately, usual treatments involve the use of medications that cause disturbances in the immune system. Thus, physicians must walk the fine line between effective therapy against the cancer and avoidance of further damage to the immune system.

Effective treatments for Kaposi's sarcoma include radiation therapy and various medications such as etoposide, vinblastine, vincristine, bleomycin, or biological agents such as interferon that have relatively mild side effects. As in antiviral trials, these studies will require large numbers of patients to draw valid conclusions about the success of treatment.

Summary

The outlook for treatment of AIDS shows early promise in several areas. The most important single objective is to prevent infection in the first place, through education, counseling, and behavior change of high-risk groups. In addition, knowledge of the molecular anatomy of the virus has contributed greatly to vaccine development. A major mystery still surrounds the exact mechanism of immune failure in AIDS, and this gap in understanding has been an obstacle to rational treatment of the immune disorder. Many effective treatments are at hand for the infections and neoplasms that complicate AIDS, but ultimate success will depend on reversing the immune deficiency. In all of these areas, we are entering an era of clinical trials that will involve rigorous, controlled studies in the pursuit of safe and effective treatment.

Medical Treatment of Kaposi's Sarcoma

Ronald Mitsuyasu, M.D.

Our brief experience with the epidemic form of Kaposi's sarcoma (KS) and AIDS has not yet yielded a consistently effective treatment for KS. We lack a clear understanding of the cause of the tumor and the mechanisms affecting the underlying immune deficiency. For the majority of patients, the opportunistic infections that occur as a result of AIDS are more of a problem than the KS tumors. However, as the functioning of the immune system worsens, the growth of the KS tumors does appear to increase. In the classic form of KS occuring in elderly Jewish men with relatively normal immune system functions, the tumor is easily controlled with local radiation therapy or chemotherapy. When KS has developed as a result of deliberate suppression of the immune system (for example, to prevent the system from rejecting a kidney transplant), the tumors disappear once the immune-suppressive drugs are stopped. The epidemic form of KS (the kind that is seen with AIDS) tends to grow more rapidly. It has not responded as well to the conventional treatments for this tumor.

Thus, researchers have developed new treatments with experimental drugs. These new treatments are aimed at stimulating the immune system to help it function properly. There are three major approaches to treatment of KS:

1. Radiotherapy. Skin lesions appear to be highly sensitive to radiotherapy (X-ray treatment). Radiation treatment with either cobalt or electron beams directed at the site of the skin lesions are the treatments of choice for such tumors. Radiation is generally successful in causing shrinkage or disappearance of tumors in the area specifically treated. It does not, however, cure the disease or affect tumors outside of the site of radiation. In the AIDS setting, when the tumor grows rapidly, radiation has been reserved primarily for the treatment of painful lesions or tumors that interfere with the function of vital organs. When lesions cause swelling of the skin, or have an obviously unsightly cosmetic effect, radiation may also be considered. A new experimental approach called "hemi-body irradiation" uses high doses of irradiation delivered to one half of the body at a time. This treatment has been used with patients who have widespread KS. Its side effects include local skin irritation from the radiation beam, some nausea, occasional mouth sores, diarrhea, and lowered blood counts in some individuals. Hemi-body irradiation has brought about shrinkage and sometimes disappearance of KS lesions, but the aggravation of underlying opportunistic infections has been a complication of this approach. Since hemi-body irradiation does not deal with the tumor on a total body basis, KS tumors may recur.

2. Chemotherapy. Chemotherapeutic agents are medications injected into the bloodstream which act to prevent the multiplication of rapidly growing cells. Cancer cells are the desired target of chemotherapy, but other rapidly growing cells are also affected, such as those that produce hair, the mucous membrane linings of the mouth and gastrointestinal tract, and blood cells (white blood cells, platelets, and red blood cells). Several chemotherapy drugs have been used in the treatment of Kaposi's sarcoma. The classic form of KS has been very sensitive and responsive to conventional treatments with drugs such as vinblastine (Velban) and actinomycin-D. In contrast, the epidemic AIDS form of KS grows more rapidly and does not respond as readily to these treatments. Furthermore, patients are more likely to develop opportunistic infections. Most AIDS patients start chemotherapy with lower than normal blood counts, and chemotherapy further affects the bone marrow's ability to produce new blood cells. Consequently, safe types and doses of chemotherapy drugs may be severely limited. For those who are able to receive chemotherapy, several drugs have been found to be helpful. Conventional drugs such as vinblastine and vincristine (Oncovin) have helped some patients. Newer, experimental agents such as VP-16 or razazone (ICRF) have also provided responses. Giving more than one chemotherapy agent at the same time (combination chemotherapy) has both benefits and disadvantages.

By using drugs in combination, which interfere differently with tumor cell growth or which act at different stages of cell reproduction, there is a higher likelihood that more tumor cells will be destroyed with one chemotherapy treatment. The disadvantage is that there are generally more side effects when combining several chemotherapy drugs.

An effective combination chemotherapy regimen presently in use includes three drugs: adriamycin, vinblastine, and bleomycin (known as ABV). Each of these drugs alone has an effect on the treatment of KS but all have side effects which include temporary lowering of blood counts, temporary hair loss, nausea, diarrhea, occasional fatigue, and fever. Many of these side effects limit the drug dose that can be safely administered. Frequent blood tests are necessary to monitor for the effects of chemotherapy on blood counts, liver and kidney function. Lowering of white blood cell counts below a certain level may allow the development of infections, which are a problem in view of the underlying immunodeficiency of AIDS. A lowered platelet count may increase the possibility of bleeding. Careful observation of these problems by both the patient and his physician may decrease the possibility of their occurrence.

As yet, there is no "best treatment" for KS with AIDS. Each approach has both advantages and disadvantages. It is possible that our present inability to restore normal immune system function will limit the effectiveness of chemotherapy in the AIDS setting.

3. Biologic Modifiers. While the goal of radiation and chemotherapy is the destruction of cancerous cells, biologic modifiers act to assist, boost, or amplify the natural body mechanisms in controlling and eliminating deviant cells. Immunotherapy is a form of biologic modification in that the desired result is strengthening natural immune system responses. Presumably, since the epidemic form of KS develops in association with immune deficiency (AIDS), it may be particularly responsive to immunotherapy. Agents such as interferon, which are capable of regulating some immune system responses as well as acting directly against viruses and tumor cells, have particular appeal as a method of treating AIDS-associated KS. Several research projects have already demonstrated the activity of interferon in shrinking and sometimes eliminating KS lesions in persons with AIDS. One form of interferon, known as alpha interferon, was found to cause as much as an overall 40 percent tumor shrinkage rate in studies conducted at the University of California Los Angeles, San Francisco General Hospital, and Memorial Sloan Kettering Hospital in New York. Side effects of interferon include fatigue and weakness, fevers, muscle aches, occasional diarrhea, and some hair loss with long-term use. Occasional recurrence of tumors has occurred despite the overall high response rate. Reduced blood counts and impaired liver function may show up in tests and can affect the amount of interferon that may be safely administered.

These results, while encouraging, are still preliminary, and further study of this agent both alone and in combination with chemotherapeutic agents will be necessary to establish its overall role in the treatment of Kaposi's sarcoma.

Other biologic modifiers which may have a direct influence on the immune system include agents such as gamma and beta interferon, interleukin 2, and various thymic hormone preparations. These drugs are currently being tested in limited fashion at selected medical research centers around the country. Their ultimate role in the treatment of KS or in improving the immune system has yet to be established.

Caution should be advised in deciding on experimental treatment approaches. Patients should seek out reputable medical oncologists (cancer specialists), preferably at university teaching hospitals where careful monitoring for side effects and thorough evaluation of the effectiveness of these agents can be established.

Choosing Alternative Therapies

Chuck Frutchey

What kind of treatment to pursue is a difficult decision for people with AIDS and ARC. After all, when you're sick, you just naturally seek some sort of treatment. But with the huge number of competing therapies, both medical and alternative, choosing one seems like a game of pin-the-tail-on-the-donkey. This problem gets larger every day as more and more people discover that they have been exposed to the AIDS virus and that they want to do something now rather than later.

Many people choose alternative therapies as their only treatment or in conjunction with medical treatments. The term "alternative therapies" refers to all types of intervention against disease that are not part of the Western medical tradition. This represents a huge range of treatments—everything from acupuncture, yoga, Chinese herbal medicines, to visualization and mega-vitamins. Many alternative therapies have a lot of success behind them, and some have a theoretical framework to explain how they work. Others are newer and seem to offer something definite, but sometimes it is difficult to separate what works from the patients' expectations, or whether success was due to chance. Some advertised therapies are very suspect or pure bunk. If you are considering using an alternative therapy, it is important to distinguish between those that may work and those that probably will not.

A major problem in evaluating alternative therapies is the lack of hard data. While many alternative therapies seem promising in the treatment of AIDS, ARC, and HIV infection, very few of these have been rigorously tested in controlled experiments. Without this kind of testing, it is impossible to be sure how much healing is due to the therapy, how much is due to the placebo effect, and how much is due to chance. Without following a group of people through a particular therapy, researchers find it impossible to determine what percent of people have benefited. However, sometimes even medical experimental drugs are given to people before their efficacy is proven. This usually happens only when a patient's condition is quite severe.

Some therapies, such as acupuncture, have a proven effect in one area (pain killing) but not in others (immune boosting). Other therapies, such as visualization, seem to work well in many situations but have yet to be studied to find what their limitations are. Clearly, there are many alternative therapies that deserve to be studied closely, but very little is being done in the way of long-term evaluations.

Selecting Therapies

A bias in favor of traditional Western medicine by health-care providers and funding sources is part of the reason for few long-term alternative studies. At the same time some alternative practitioners have been reluctant to engage in rigorous testing and evaluations of their own methods. In fact, many alternative therapists* say it is unfair to give some patients a placebo in a controlled study. And yet many people face the choice of an alternative therapy without knowing whether it is helpful or useless. It is almost impossible to know about all the therapies, what they purport to do, and how effective they are. A more practical solution is to have some guidelines and questions that are good for any therapy you may be considering. The guidelines that are discussed here were developed mainly for evaluating alternative, non-medical therapies, but most of the considerations apply to your medical doctor and drug therapies as well.

---

*Therapist is defined in this article as a "person who is trained in methods and treatment other than the use of drugs or surgery." (Webster's)

The first step is to see a doctor. Even if you decide to pursue an alternative therapy, there is no substitute for consulting with a doctor who can monitor your vital signs, blood work, etc. Any alternative practitioner who tells you to stay away from physicians should make you immediately suspicious. If your medical doctor advises you not to try anything alternative, you should question that advice as well. It is important for different care-givers to communicate with each other so they do not do things that will contradict each other. Your doctor and your herbalist may be giving you medications that can react with each other and put you in danger. If each knows what the other is doing, dangerous situations can be avoided. Your medical record is usually the most complete description of your health and disease history; it is therefore useful to have your alternative treatments recorded there as well.

If you decide that you would like to pursue an alternative therapy, you need to do some research. [Editor's note: the AIDS organization in your area will likely be able to provide you with listings of local alternative practitioners. See the listing of AIDS organizations in the resource directory in Section Ten.] Health food stores are also a good place to find referrals. Ask friends or acquaintances about what they have heard of or what they recommend. Collect as much information as you think you need before you make a choice. You may decide to pursue more than one therapy at a time, but, again, make sure that the different practitioners talk to each other.

Selecting an Alternative Practitioner

After you decide on the therapy you want, there are several important considerations in choosing a care-giver. First, know who your care-giver is, his or her reputation, and how long this therapy has been a specialty. Are there any colleagues with the same specialty who will give a good reference? Is it possible to talk to previous clients about the quality of care? If the therapist is unknown and can provide no references, look for another. Also find out if the therapist has done any previous work with people who have AIDS or ARC.

The next consideration is whether the care-giver can explain the therapy to you in a way that makes sense to you. Is he or she eager to answer your questions or willing to talk to your doctor or other care-givers? What is the underlying philosophy from which the therapist operates? If you get explanations that sound more like gibberish than reasoned thought, you should think twice about whether to trust this person with your health.

Another related concern is whether the therapy seems to make sense to you. Does it fit in with your own philosophy? Can you believe in it? Does it seem more like hype than healing? Some alternative therapies maintain that belief in the effectiveness of the therapy is a major part of how it works; so if you don't believe, you may be wasting your time.

Also, be aware of the placebo effect. Approximately 30 percent of people pursuing any therapy will show some improvement just because they believe that something good is being done for them. If someone tells you that one-third of people on therapy X improved, realize that it may not be significant.

You should also ask for any available documentation on the therapy you are considering. How many people have done this therapy? How many have gotten better? By how much? What about those who did not get better? By how much? Are there any side effects? Are there possible cross reactions with other drugs or conditions? Does the therapist take a complete history before and after therapy? Are adequate records being kept? Has this therapy been used for AIDS and ARC before? Has any of this data improved understanding of how this therapy works? Therapists who insist on faith and spurn data are likely going to be a waste of your time and money.

There are several things you should do while you are receiving therapy. Monitor yourself by keeping a log or notes. The therapist should be doing this, too, but keep your own records to compare. If you are not feeling better or showing some improvement after what seems to you like a reasonable time, then ask your therapist about it.

Not all therapies work for everyone. Continue to ask questions and be a part of the therapy, not just a passive recipient. Stop the therapy if you think it is useless or harming you. Make sure you are not going broke. Don't sacrifice your rent and food money for your treatment. Most practitioners will make some financial arrangement that is workable for you.

Exploring alternatives will not hurt you. Keep an open mind and realize that there is more than one way to get well. There is much truth and good healing in alternative therapies that cannot be currently explained, but neither can they be denied. What *can* hurt you, however, is chasing after cures without a critical eye. Just accepting the effectiveness of a therapy on faith is a good way to get taken advantage of or get sicker, or both.

Be clear when you start a new therapy about what you expect to gain and how you will know when you are better. Getting well is possible with AIDS and ARC, and it is important to know that it can happen for you. But the old adage still applies: buyer beware.

Section Five

Prevention: A Socio-Sexual Perspective

CAUTION: SEXUALLY EXPLICIT MATERIAL. *NOT* READING THIS MAY BE HAZARDOUS TO YOUR HEALTH!

Having AIDS does not have to mean giving up sex, but it does mean some changes in attitude, approach, and activity. The process of such change can contribute to the expansion of sexual pleasure, emotional growth, and the satisfaction of being able to adapt. It can lead to development of more intimate and satisfying relationships with others.

"Expressions of Sexuality"

Prevention

AIDS Safe-Sex Guidelines

Is It Safe to Have Unsafe Sex with My Partner?

AIDS Doesn't Discriminate

Women and AIDS: Risks and Concerns

Alcohol, Drugs, and AIDS

Expressions of Sexuality

Prevention

How Is Aids Contagious?

This answer requires some understanding of general principles that apply to all contagious diseases. In general, disease transmission requires a vehicle carrying a significant number of germs into a susceptible person. A vehicle can be microscopic amounts of blood such as in the case of some types of hepatitis. It can be urine or semen in the case of cytomegalovirus (CMV). It can be pus or stool or the objects contaminated with these. Not all germs are present in all body fluids or secretions.

How Are We Susceptible to Infections?

We are susceptible either by (1) exposure to very invasive germs that respect none of the natural barriers most people have, or (2) damage to natural barriers allowing invasion of germs that otherwise might not have a chance to cause infection.

What Are Our Natural Barriers?

Intact skin and mucous membranes of the nose, throat, urethra, and rectum. Stomach acid, which kills many swallowed germs. Healthy cells of the nose and lungs, which can filter and expel inhaled germs. Normal mucus and saliva production, which can coat and "neutralize" many germs.

Are There Any Other Barriers?

A hand can be held over the mouth when coughing, a tissue or handkerchief can be held over the mouth when sneezing. A condom can be used when having sexual intercourse. Any means of avoiding direct contact with the excretions and secretions (urine, stool, blood, semen, saliva) of other persons represent barriers that limit the chance for you to acquire germs those people may harbor—even if they don't appear ill.

You Mean I Can Catch an Infection from Someone Who Does Not Appear Ill?

Yes. Many infections are contagious even during the "incubation period." During the time after a person is infected but before he or she feels sick, the germ for that illness may be transmitted to other people. The incubation period for AIDS may be from seven months to six years. Thus, there may be two years or more between the time the person is infected and feels sick with AIDS. [Editor's note: Further research suggests that the incubation period may be as long as ten years; researchers believe once exposed, individuals are infected with the AIDS virus for life.] It is therefore possible and probable (but not proven) that the AIDS virus may be spread during this time.

Sex and AIDS

Reducing risk for AIDS may mean making changes in sexual practices, but it does not mean denying the sexual part of one's life. Fear of AIDS can and probably will stir homophobic responses in many of us. Sex and intimacy may be seen as bad and to be avoided at a time when we need more intimacy and self-affirmation. We may need to create a kind and rational "parent" in our heads that counteracts such negative thoughts and guides us toward a healthy regard for our bodies and the bodies of those we love. We urge careful considerations of the following points and their implied suggestions.

There are general factors agreed upon by virtually all researchers as representing significant risk: (1) Sexual activity in which bodily secretions are exchanged; (2) the more partners with whom sexual activity includes secretion exchange, the greater the risk; (3) the injection of illicit drugs or the shared use of needles for such injections, and by logical extension, sexual contact with those known to use drugs intravenously.

AIDS Safe-Sex Guidelines

Remember: *ANY activity which allows for possible contact between the body fluids or feces of one person and the mouth, anus, vagina, bloodstream, cuts, or sores of another person is considered UNSAFE at this time.*

SAFE-SEX PRACTICES

- Massage, hugging, body-to-body rubbing
- Dry social kissing
- Masturbation (touching your own genitals)
- Acting out sexual fantasies (that do not include any unsafe sex practices)
- Using vibrators or other sex toys (provided you only use your own)

LOW-RISK SEX PRACTICES

These activities are not considered completely safe.

- French (wet) kissing (to be avoided if either partner has mouth sores)
- Mutual masturbation, touching each other's genitals (Risk may be further reduced by using disposable latex gloves to guard against cuts on hands.)
- Vaginal or anal intercourse using a condom
- Oral sex, male (*fellatio*) using a condom
- Oral sex, female (*cunnilingus*), using a thin piece of latex between the mouth and the female organ (Risk is increased during menstruation.)
- EXTERNAL contact with semen or urine (*watersports*) provided there are no breaks in the skin

UNSAFE-SEX PRACTICES

- Vaginal or anal intercourse without a condom
- Semen, urine or feces in the mouth or vagina
- Unprotected oral sex (*fellatio or cunnilingus*)
- Unprotected penetration of vagina or anus with hand or finger
- Oral-anal contact (*rimming*) or anal penetration with fist (*fisting*)
- Blood contact of any kind
- Sharing sex toys or needles

Certain sexual practices are known to be associated with an increased risk of sexually transmitted disease. Unless you *and* your partner have been exclusively monogamous for seven years or more, following safe-sex guidelines is advised. These practices decrease your risk of AIDS. *Remember* the principles of protective barriers that block the spread of germs in blood, secretions, and excretions from person to person.

Is It Safe to Have Unsafe Sex with My Partner?

Many people have the mistaken idea that unsafe sex with a partner is safe, especially if the relationship is monogamous. That is rarely true. For most of us, it is too risky to have unsafe sex during the AIDS epidemic. Nearly all of the publicity about AIDS has focused on avoiding unsafe sex with multiple partners. That is because from an epidemiological point of view, unsafe sex with multiple partners spreads AIDS far more widely than unsafe sex with a single partner. Monogamous relationships do cut down on the spread of AIDS, but they don't guarantee the safety of the persons in the relationships. No one knows for certain just how much re-exposure to the virus is required for the disease to result. The body's defenses may be able to resist some quantity of the virus, but at some point, if you continue to be exposed (even to viruses from the same person), your body's defenses may be overcome. It is not safe to have unsafe sex with your lover (or anyone else), UNLESS:

1) You have *both* been in an *exclusively* monogamous relationship with each other for at least seven years or more *and* neither of you has shared IV needles, had transfusions, or used other blood products; or

2) You have both been tested for HIV antibodies twice over a six-month period and have both received negative test results and haven't since been exposed.

Caring about your partner these days means protecting one another from re-exposure to the virus. Try new and safer ways of sexual expression. Use condoms if you have sex. Avoid unsafe sex. Take care of one another. There is nothing you can do about the past. There is a great deal you can do about the future. If you would like more information or assistance, help is available. (Contact your local AIDS organization.)

AIDS Doesn't Discriminate

Contrary to what most people believe, AIDS isn't just a disease of the gay community. AIDS is just a disease. And like all diseases, it began somewhere and moved into one population, on to another, and it's now on its way to others. However, regardless of what population you're in, AIDS can be avoided. Because every day we're learning more and more how AIDS is spread. And it doesn't have to do with your sex or sexual orientation. It has to do with whom you have sex (male or female) and what type of sexual acts you practice. There are guidelines to follow. It is important that all sexually active people understand them:

1. **Communicate with Your Sexual Partner.** Find out your partner's past sexual activity and decide whether you want to have sex with this person, and what type of sex you want to practice.

2. **Limit Your Number of Sexual Partners.** Simply, the fewer people you have sex with, the fewer chances you're taking.

3. **Identify the High-Risk Groups.** Any male who has had sexual contact with another male, intravenous drug users, hemophiliacs, or any sexual partner of the above since 1977, falls into the high-risk category.

Portions of the article are reprinted from "A Special Appeal to People of Color," and "A Special Appeal to People Over 45," by the San Francisco AIDS Foundation.

4. **Adopt Safe-Sex Practices.** As we said earlier, AIDS can be avoided by following safe-sex guidelines. AIDS doesn't make choices. It is a serious, growing problem for the entire population. FIGHT THE FEAR WITH THE FACTS.

A SPECIAL APPEAL TO PEOPLE OF COLOR

Some people have the mistaken notion that AIDS is mainly a "white man's disease"—that people of color aren't much at risk for AIDS. The statistics prove otherwise. In the United States, roughly four out of every ten people with AIDS are non-white. Twenty-five percent of Americans with AIDS are black. Nearly 15 percent are Hispanic. The AIDS virus does not discriminate on the basis of race, age, gender, or sexual orientation. AIDS can strike anyone who engages in the activities that can spread AIDS—unsafe sex or the sharing of IV drug needles. The only way we have of limiting this epidemic is through prevention. If we as a community are going to survive this epidemic, all of us need to eliminate unsafe sex and needle-sharing from our lifestyles until a cure or vaccine for AIDS is available. No one has ever died from the frustration of giving up a few unsafe sex practices. Far too many have died of AIDS. Together we can stop the spread of this disease.

A SPECIAL APPEAL TO PEOPLE OVER FORTY-FIVE

Some people have the mistaken notion that AIDS is a young person's disease—that older people aren't at great risk of contracting AIDS. The statistics indicate otherwise. There are cases of AIDS among newborn babies and cases of AIDS among people in their eighties. AIDS does not discriminate on the basis of age, race, gender, or sexual orientation. In San Francisco, 35 percent of people with AIDS are over forty. Nearly 10 percent of San Francisco AIDS cases are found in people fifty and older. By contrast, only 15 percent of people with AIDS here are in their twenties.

Studies conducted for the San Francisco AIDS Foundation by a professional research firm indicate that people over forty-five in San Francisco, compared to any other demographic group, tend to be less knowledgeable about AIDS prevention, and more likely to engage in anonymous unsafe sex than their younger counterparts. We urge people over forty-five to reassess their risk of contracting AIDS and to help spread the word to their contemporaries: People over forty-five are definitely at risk for AIDS.

Help *is* available. STOP AIDS projects in San Francisco and Los Angeles offer one-evening discussion groups about the AIDS epidemic for people of all ages. Remember, with AIDS it's the sexual activity you engage in that counts, not how old you are. Please protect yourself and your partners from AIDS.

Women and AIDS: Risks and Concerns

Nancy Stoller Shaw, Ph.D.

AIDS is a women's health issue. In the United States, about eight percent of people with AIDS are women. As of May 1986, over 1300 women had been diagnosed with AIDS and as many as 25,000 women may be infected with the virus that causes AIDS. Hundreds of children have been infected with the virus, either through transmission at birth or from blood products received before 1985. In addition, many women's facilities and friends have been personally affected by the epidemic.

AIDS can affect all communities; no age, income level, or ethnic group is immune. So far, of the women who have AIDS, 50 percent have been black, 23 percent have been Latina, and 27 percent have been white. A small number of Asian and Native American women have also contracted AIDS.

How Do Women Get AIDS?

The Five Risk Categories:

1. National data show that the most prevalent risk category for women is IV-drug use (50 percent). These women have contracted the virus through sharing needles or other drug paraphernalia.

2. The second risk category is high-risk sexual acts between men and women. In absolute numbers, 244 women were in this category in May 1986. Even though many more men than women have AIDS, heterosexual contact was the suspected route of infection for only fifty-seven men.

Why do more women than men appear to develop AIDS after heterosexual contacts? One explanation is that there are more infected men than there are infected women. This means that in terms of heterosexual contact, more men are capable of transmitting the virus. A second theory is that while semen is a proven route of AIDS viral transmission, the virus has been found in only minute amounts in vaginal secretions. Some heterosexual contact includes anal intercourse, an important risk factor for viral transmission. Research on the relationship of different types of heterosexual activity and viral transmission is just beginning. Research data shows that 72 percent of women with AIDS have had male partners who use IV drugs; another 19 percent of the women had bisexual men as sex partners.

3. The third risk category for women is "transfusions with blood or blood products." This category accounts for 10 percent of all women with AIDS. New cases from earlier transfusions will continue to appear; but since 1985, the risk of transfusion-related transmission has dropped to near zero.

4. A fourth risk category for women is "hemophiliac/coagulation disorder." In May 1986, there were four adult women in this category. A few women do have coagulation disorders (a blood clotting problem) for which they receive the same types of blood products as are prescribed for hemophiliacs. As with transfusions, the current risk associated with blood products is essentially zero.

5. Finally, a significant number of women with AIDS, 20 percent of the total, cannot be linked with any route of transmission. In the Centers for Disease Control (CDC) statistics, they are referred to as "none/other."

Who are these women? For many of them, the most likely route of infection was heterosexual contact with a man who was infected with the virus but who was not in an identified risk group. His infection may have resulted from sexual contact with a person whom he did not know to be in a risk category (for example, his wife, who had a blood transfusion prior to his meeting her).

Some women were diagnosed late in their illness. This can happen when health-care providers were unaware that their female clients may have been exposed to the AIDS virus, or when a woman unexpectedly suffers a fatal bout of pneumocystis carinii pneumonia (PCP) or another opportunistic infection linked to AIDS. Such late diagnoses make it difficult to obtain adequate sex, blood, and drug histories from the patients. Thus, these women are often placed in the "other" category.

What About Artificial Insemination?

To date, no cases of AIDS have been traced to donor insemination. Four women in Australia developed antibodies to the virus after they were accidentally inseminated by an intra-uterine technique with semen from a man who was already infected. None of the women became pregnant as a result of the inseminations. Since current antibody screening programs for semen donors in the U.S. are now more stringent than even those used by the blood banks, there is almost no risk of AIDS exposure for women receiving sperm from a licensed sperm bank.

What About Lesbian Sex?

A woman who only has sex with other women is at low risk in terms of her sexual activity. There are no proven cases of viral transmission through woman-to-woman sexual contact. There are cases of lesbians getting AIDS from each other and from non-lesbians through *sharing IV needles*. And lesbians have gotten AIDS from blood transfusions. A bisexual woman who has sex with both men and women is at risk with the man if he is carrying the virus. These women should carefully follow safe-sex guidelines for reducing their risk in these cases.

In summary, the women who are at most risk of getting AIDS are those who:

- share or borrow needles or any other paraphernalia when using IV drugs;
- have sexual partners who use, or have used, IV drugs;
- have sexual partners who are bisexual men.

There is a slight risk if the woman or her partner received blood or blood products between 1977 and 1985.

The women with the least risk of contracting AIDS are those who:

- have been celibate and have received no blood products since 1977;
- have been in a completely monogamous (both partners) relationship with a man or woman since 1977;
- have only had sexual partners without any risk since 1977.

How Can Women Avoid AIDS?

The first way to avoid AIDS is to prevent exposure to the virus which causes the illness. Women can avoid AIDS by not sharing IV-drug use equipment (needles, syringes, spoons) and by not having unprotected sex.

For most sexual activity—vaginal intercourse, anal intercourse, and fellatio—the major AIDS transmission risk is from semen entering the body. The best prevention method is to use condoms (rubbers). Recent research indicates that condoms do block the AIDS virus. Condoms can be used in any kind of intercourse and in fellatio by mutual agreement—or, in fact, even without it. Of course, it is important to remember that condoms are not 100 percent effective. Women have been known to get pregnant even when using condoms as contraception.

Unprotected anal intercourse has been shown to be the most dangerous form of sexual activity when it comes to transmitting the AIDS virus. If there is a risk that the woman's partner may be carrying the virus, this activity should be avoided in all situations.

Unprotected vaginal intercourse can also lead to viral transmission, infection, and subsequent illness. During intercourse the virus could enter the woman's bloodstream through minor abrasions in the vagina or through the uterine wall or fallopian tubes after passing through the cervix. Women who have abrasions or infections which cause sores or raw areas in the vagina, or on the cervix, may be at special risk because the virus may have more direct route to the bloodstream.

Researchers have not studied the risk associated with having semen in the mouth and with swallowing semen. Since most people who engage in oral sex also engage in other sexual activities, it is difficult to separate the risk of oral sex from the other activities. However, both physicians and researchers agree that no one should swallow semen if there is a chance that it contains the virus. (When a person is infected with the AIDS virus, large amounts are found in the blood and semen. Small amounts are found in the saliva, tears, sweat, breast milk, and vaginal secretions.)

Women who wish to have unprotected sex (any sexual activity in which semen enters the body) should first be certain that their partner is not carrying the virus. The first step may be to talk with the potential partners. Partners can share their sexual histories. Talking about sex can be difficult, even when AIDS is not an issue; and there are many reasons why people keep secrets about their pasts. Also, many people are unaware of the sexual histories of their former partners. Consequently, talking does not always provide either partner with complete confidence.

In some cases, an AIDS antibody test can resolve anxiety about AIDS exposure. In other cases, neither conversation nor the antibody test is feasible or sufficient. At these times, the woman may wish to protect herself by following special protective procedures, which are often referred to as safe sex.

The most important form of protection for a woman is to prevent entry of semen into her body. If a woman chooses to have intercourse, the best form of protection is to use a condom and a spermicide containing nonoxynol-9, an ingredient that kills the AIDS virus on contact. However, nonoxynol-9 alone is not sufficient protection; a condom must be used as well. Nonoxynol-9 lubricants can be applied both inside and outside a condom. Some condoms are also pre-lubricated with spermicide. Using a condom appropriately (without breakage) will prevent the virus from entering her body during ejaculation. Whether intercourse is vaginal, anal, or oral, a condom is the most effective protective device. (**Note:** Diaphragms do *not* provide a barrier to the virus. They are effective in preventing pregnancy only because they hold the spermicides which kill the semen as it is about to enter the uterus.)

Previous exposure and current sexual activity are two separate factors. If two people are very high-risk because of their previous practices, they can still engage in very safe sexual activities.

Transmission can also occur when sex toys are shared. A woman should not share or borrow any item (dildo, or vibrator, for example) which has been used internally by a partner at risk, unless it has been thoroughly cleaned with bleach, alcohol, or hydrogen peroxide and then rinsed with water.

Can Women Transmit AIDS to Others?

Women can transmit the virus directly in four ways:

- through shared needles or equipment associated with IV-drug use;
- via sexual activity (involving vaginal secretions, menstrual blood, or rectal blood;

- during pregnancy, perinatally, or at birth;
- through lactation (breastfeeding).

Sexual Transmission. Female-to-male sexual transmission of the AIDS virus has been the focus of much attention and debate. As the data indicate, AIDS is apparently more difficult to transmit from women to men than vice-versa. However, in women who are infected, menstrual blood, rectal blood, and vaginal secretions all contain the virus. If these fluids are transmitted to the partner's bloodstream, there is a possibility of infection.

In terms of vaginal secretions and/or menstrual blood, some researchers theorize that transmission might occur during vaginal intercourse if the fluids pass into the male partner's body via the urethra or penile abrasions or sores. Some researchers believe that the higher rates of female-to-male transmission reported in central Africa may be the result of genital sores caused by malnutrition and poor health care for both men and women.

A woman's rectal blood can also transmit the virus to her sex partner. Such transmission could occur if blood were ingested during oral sex. Also, after anal sex, blood might be on the penis and then be accidentally ingested afterwards. In some studies, as many as one-third of women who have multiple sex partners report that they have engaged in anal sex in the past few years. Sometimes such activity is practiced as a means of birth control. For AIDS prevention, unprotected anal sex should never be practiced if a partner is at risk or if the partner's risk status cannot be determined.

Maternal Transmission. The transmission of the AIDS virus from infected mothers to infants, either *in utero* or perinatally, has been well established. Infection in the infants can occur without any symptoms or it can cause a variety or problems and disorders, including AIDS. It is not known what proportion of infants exposed *in utero* or perinatally will become infected and what proportion of infected infants will develop actual diseases. As of May 1986, 219 infants born to mothers at risk, or with AIDS, had developed AIDS themselves. This total does not include the many infants with AIDS-related complex (ARC) or those with positive antibody test results. Researchers agree that the total of unreported cases is much higher.

Recent preliminary data indicates that some maternal transmission occurs at delivery. Consequently, some physicians are considering the use of Caesarean section as a way of preventing transmission. Much more research is needed to understand these maternal transmission issues.

The AIDS virus has also been cultured from breast milk. There is one reported case in Australia of viral transmission from mother to infant from breast milk. In this case, the mother received a transfusion after the birth of her baby. She then nursed the baby frequently for over six months, without realizing she was infected.

How Can an Infected Woman Avoid Transmitting AIDS?

To prevent passage of the virus from a woman to her sexual partner, the woman should:

- have her male partners use condoms and herself use nonoxynol-9 during vaginal and anal sex;
- not allow her partner to have oral contact with her vaginal secretions, menstrual blood, or rectal area.

A woman can prevent maternal transmission of the virus by testing before her pregnancy. The CDC, as well as many health departments, recommend that women who may be carrying the virus be tested for antibodies prior to becoming pregnant. Many authorities strongly recommend postponement of pregnancy if the test result is positive.

A pregnant women who discovers that she is infected has several options. She may choose to terminate the pregnancy, or, if she chooses to continue it, she should be aware of the risk of AIDS viral transmission to her infant. Because little is known about prevention of maternal transmission via placental or delivery routes, the woman should obtain care from an obstetric-pediatric team that is knowledgeable about AIDS.

A woman who is infected with the virus should not ordinarily nurse her child. However, for those women who are healthy and only "at risk," pediatricians recommend that breastfeeding be encouraged because the immunological protections outweigh the risk of transmission.

AIDS: Special Concerns for Women

While there are some ways that AIDS is the same illness for women as it is for men, there are also some very important ways in which it is different. First, women get different illnesses from men. Men, and especially the gay men that presently make up the bulk of AIDS cases, are much more likely than women to contract the cancer called Kaposi's sarcoma (KS). In some cases, KS will develop very slowly over a three- to five-year period. Women are more likely to contract one of the opportunistic infections, such as PCP. The illnesses that affect women are often those which are severely incapacitating and have a serious short-term prognosis in terms of fatality rates.

Second, women get pregnant. Women who are infected and pregnant sometimes need special care to prevent their health from deteriorating more rapidly since a woman's immune system is depressed during pregnancy. Pregnancy can accelerate the course of illnesses associated with AIDS and ARC and perhaps also the underlying disease syndrome itself. Women who are already ill and discover they are pregnant need information both about the potential impact of pregnancy on their own health and maternal-fetal transmission.

A third aspect of AIDS that is unique to women is the female social role of mothering. From this role flow two important consequences. First, when a woman becomes ill with AIDS or ARC, her role as caretaker for the child or children or for other adults in the household is immediately affected. The family is severely disrupted, and each family member will have to make many adjustments. A mother's children may be indirectly affected by her diagnosis; for example, the children may be forbidden to go to school. The mother must cope with her own life-threatening illness while she must also deal with the impact of AIDS on her family. Demographic studies show that many of the women at risk for AIDS have young children; these women are often the sole support of these children.

Another consequence of the social role of motherhood is the care for a child with AIDS. With AIDS, as with other sicknesses, the mother must often assume primary care for the child. But since 75 percent of all pediatric AIDS cases are currently the result of maternal transmission, the mother herself may be ill. Her illness and responsibility may be complicated further by incarceration, poor health, and the threat of foster care proceedings. If the mother is healthy enough to care for her child, she must still cope with the complex issues of medical and home care, school access, friends, and family stress.

At the 1985 International Conference on AIDS in Atlanta, many researchers discussing sexuality referred to "sexually active" men and "promiscuous" women. Prostitutes were described as a "reservoir of infections." Just as gay men are stigmatized for their sexual activity, so too are women who cannot prove that they contracted the virus from their husbands or from blood transfusions. AIDS is a serious disease that affects many people from different backgrounds; efforts to prevent AIDS and help people with the disease are only hampered by the use of inappropriate and inaccurate stereotypes.

Resources for Women

Because the total number of women infected with the AIDS virus is much smaller than the number of infected men, the resources available for women are much more limited.

Women need targeted AIDS services designed to meet their specific needs. Many AIDS organizations have only begun to develop women's support groups; many have only recently recognized the need to hire and train staff who are sensitive to women's issues. Many women with AIDS are from poor backgrounds; as a result, they may need expanded services during their illness.

Resources and services for people with AIDS must also address ethnic concerns and issues. Over 70 percent of all female AIDS cases are black or Latina women. Special outreach efforts will be needed in many communities. Working with local ethnic health and civic organizations can be an important step in raising community awareness of AIDS and of its prevention.

Women as Health-Care Providers

From the very beginning of the AIDS epidemic, women have played primary roles in the care of people with the disease. As health-care providers—doctors, nurses, social workers, technicians, counselors, as well as the many mothers who care for their sons or daughters—women have contributed greatly to our understanding of how to offer supportive, safe, and effective care to people with AIDS. These contributions are frequently recognized by individuals—patients, their friends, and families—but often this important role of women has been bypassed by administrators, medical institutions, and the media.

Women in both the lesbian and heterosexual communities have also helped to develop support networks for people with AIDS. Women deserve and need support, official appreciation, and recognition. AIDS presents many challenges and risks to both men and women. An effective response must recognize the similarities and the differences in needs, at-risk behavior, and socio-economic status of women as well as of men.

Alcohol, Drugs, and AIDS

There is growing evidence of a significant connection between AIDS and alcohol and drug abuse. Substance abuse is an issue we can no longer afford to ignore. Drugs and alcohol don't cause AIDS. AIDS is caused by a virus. But there are at least three ways in which alcohol and drugs can increase your chances of getting AIDS.

First, alcohol and drugs depress the immune system and make you more susceptible to disease. Alcohol, marijuana, speed, cocaine, poppers, and other recreational chemicals lower your resistance to disease. In some research studies, poppers have been implicated in increasing the risk of KS (Kaposi's sarcoma). Drugs and alcohol weaken your health, increase stress rather than relieve it, and help the AIDS virus overcome your body's defenses.

Second, alcohol and drugs reduce your ability to stick to judgments about what's safe and what isn't. Studies demonstrate a strong correlation between alcohol and drug use and unsafe-sex practices.

Third, sharing IV-drug needles transmits the AIDS virus directly from the bloodstream of one infected person to the bloodstream of another. If you do take the risk of using IV drugs, *don't* share needles! It's a direct route for the transmission of AIDS. There are thousands of IV-drug users in America

This article was originally published by the San Francisco AIDS Foundation and funded by the San Francisco Department of Public Health.

with AIDS, and probably thousands of others who are still incubating the virus and who are contagious. *Don't share needles!* According to experts who treat substance abuse we have had a major epidemic of substance abuse in our country for years—so much so that most of us have accepted substance abuse as a routine part of life. What was once routine, however, is now deadly.

Remember:

- Sharing needles is dangerous. Don't share needles.

- Alcohol and drugs depress the immune system. Protect your health.

- Getting high can lead to practicing unsafe-sex and exposure (or re-exposure) to the AIDS virus.

Now is the perfect time to take a fresh look at your own use of alcohol and drugs—and to get some help (often free) to find out if you have a drinking or drug problem that may increase your chances of getting AIDS.

Expressions of Sexuality

Rex Reece, Ph.D.

General Purposes of Sex

Sex satiates a combination of physical and emotional needs—different needs for different people at different times. Among other things, sexual desire may include a need for physical release, emotional expression and intimacy, reassurance of being loved or of being desirable. Sex can also be a way of passing time, the result of habit, or an escape from any number of uncomfortable feelings. For a person with AIDS, physical intimacy—a term that includes warm sex (expressions of affection and pleasure such as touching, holding, stroking, caressing, and endearing comments) and/or hot sex (passion, desire, physical arousal, and perhaps orgasm)—can continue to be an expression of the feelings and needs that have always been a part of his/her sexuality. Bear in mind that just as personal motivations for sex are based on a variety of needs, the means to respond may be equally varied. Finding alternate activities to meet these needs can be helpful.

AIDS Effect on Sexual Desire

Physical illness can alter one's needs for sex. Health problems may contribute to one's feelings of loneliness and isolation and, therefore, increase the need for reassurance of love and care from others. AIDS sometimes causes visible physical changes that can make a person with AIDS feel less sexually desirable. Some people with AIDS may become more physically dependent as a result of their illness, and consequently may feel unneeded or burdensome. Physical intimacy can help combat these and other uncomfortable feelings for someone with AIDS. Safe sex can reassure a person with AIDS that it is still possible to give pleasure to another person or, perhaps more importantly, to receive pleasure.

Illness can make *anyone* less interested in sex and sometimes less physically responsive. When one does not feel well, whether physically or emotionally, it is not unusual to be less interested in sex. Certainly, many medications affect sexual interest and response. Furthermore, because AIDS has some association with sexual activity, a person with AIDS may be less interested in sex because of anger, guilt, frustration, or fear involved in that association. The risk of transmission to others or one's increased vulnerability to other infections may significantly inhibit one's sexual desire or activity. Even when the desire is there, the physical response may be altered. Physical stamina may be lessened so that one has limited energy; sexual sessions may be somewhat shorter or less active than during pre-illness times. Men may experience less frequent erections or have difficulty maintaining them; for women, lubrication may not be as abundant or orgasms may not be as readily forthcoming.

Changing Sexual Behavior and Attitudes

Limitations are often frustrating, and reading a list of AIDS do's and don'ts is probably no exception. Don't let the safe-sex guidelines contribute to a sense of futility. Keep in mind that the list of precautions and prohibitions is specific and finite; the "do not" list is much shorter than the list of what is safe and possible to enjoy. Focus on what you can do, be positive, and enjoy it.

How many people have rather limited views of what sex is? For example, for some it is restricted to something like arousal, insertion, and, finally, climax. For others, sexual play may follow a different routine. As a result of AIDS, some people will take the opportunity to develop additional and varied intimate interactions that are satisfying.

One *can* change attitudes and behavior. Many of the specifics of how one likes to have sex or make love are *learned;* what excites an individual today may differ considerably from what was especially enjoyable in previous years. For example, many people can remember that the idea of orally stimulating a partner's genitals was at first repulsive, yet it may have become a favorite sexual activity. Perhaps, with some time and repeated experiences, it may be possible to develop such erotic associations with condoms and other practices which have obvious health benefits.

These examples suggest that it *is* possible to develop new ways of enjoying sex unless pride, fear, anger, or some other emotional resistances, block experimentation. Adapting and experimenting will be more difficult for some because of the sexual guilt and inhibitions that most people have internalized in our society, regardless of how sexually active one has been or how creative one may have been in past sexual behavior. Some persons with AIDS will be able to accommodate this unfortunate and difficult situation and achieve surprising new levels of sexual satisfaction.

It is easier to make these changes if one can talk somewhat comfortably and openly about sex. This process could begin by voicing one's needs for physical intimacy while acknowledging the fears regarding transmission of AIDS or the vulnerability of one's own health related to that exposure. Even though previously one may have been uncomfortable with such questions as "What do you like to do in bed?," some discussion of "What can we safely do?" or "Let's try...," may now be necessary in order to feel safe, avoid transmission, and be physically prepared with preventative supplies like condoms. Talking openly about the frustrations and disappointments when things do not work out the way one had hoped is often helpful. The experience of making all the necessary preparations and taking precautions with someone—sometimes awkward, inhibiting, embarrassing, frustrating, sad, or funny—can increase affection between two people and, in turn, can be especially reassuring for someone who is seriously ill.

The need for physical intimacy is great; so is the concern about transmission. Aspects of previous sexual patterns will be missed, some more than others. Changing sexual patterns and habits is difficult, but for most persons with AIDS it is necessary for his/her own safety and the health of others. Because of AIDS, sex is not likely to be what it was before; but with the full knowledge and cooperation of one's partner and openness to new experiences, satisfying sex and intimate pleasures can be achieved.

Having AIDS does not have to mean giving up sex, but it does mean some changes in attitude, approach, and activity. The process of such change can contribute to the expansion of sexual pleasure, emotional growth, and the satisfaction of being able to adapt. It can lead to development of more intimate and satisfying relationships with others.

Section Six

A Self-Care Perspective

The guidelines for home care and symptom management enabled me to care for my son with AIDS at home until the last moments of his life. Without this practical information, I couldn't have done it.

— A mother of an AIDS patient

Nutrition and Exercise

Dental Care

General Hygiene Measures and Risk Reduction

Home Care

Symptom Management

Managing the Side Effects of Treatment for Kaposi's Sarcoma

Nutrition and Exercise

Jennifer Lang, R.N., M.N.

Nutritional concerns are crucial for the self-care of persons with AIDS and ARC and also for those with HIV infection. Fevers and infections create an increased metabolic rate and an increased need for protein and calorie intake, but diarrhea and loss of appetite make it difficult to meet such increased nutritional needs. Poor nutrition may also contribute further to suppression of cell-mediated immunity; many scientific studies have shown that protein-calorie malnutrition reduces the numbers and effectiveness of circulating lymphocytes (cells). Maintaining an optimal nutritional state will not cure AIDS, but it could influence positively the numbers and function of lymphocytes and it could boost resistance to opportunistic infections.

Protein is essential to produce new cells and repair damaged tissues whenever the body experiences stress, as occurs when fighting infections. When this need for protein cannot be met through dietary intake, the body breaks down muscle tissue and recycles these muscle proteins (the "building blocks of life") into new production and tissue formation. The body is more likely to steal proteins from muscles which are not being used. Therefore, inactivity as well as poor protein-calorie intake and infection all contribute to the "wasting" syndrome so commonly seen in AIDS. In order to prevent muscle deterioration, it is important that both nutrition and exercise receive equal attention.

How Do I Meet My Nutritional Needs?

Healthy people who are not stressed by infection or increased activity need daily intake of about 2700 calories and 56 grams of protein for men and 2000 calories and 45 grams of protein for women just to maintain their weight. During an illness such as AIDS, the requirement increases to as much as 5000 calories per day. A good rule of thumb is to try for 50 calories per kilogram of ideal body weight (1 kilogram equals 2.2 pounds; for example, 175 pounds equals 79.5 kilograms) and for 1.5 grams of protein per kilogram. For a 155 pound (70 kg.) man this would be 3500 calories per day with 105 grams of protein. In addition to protein and calories, it is important to maintain a well-balanced diet which will supply minerals, vitamins, and other elements. These supplements to the diet can be accomplished by choosing foods from each of the four basic food groups. Multivitamin supplements are recommended in moderation and after consultation with a physician.

What Are the Basic Four Food Groups?

Fruit and Vegetable Group. Four servings a day of salad, cooked vegetables, raw or cooked fruits or juices supply needed vitamins and minerals. A serving can consist of one-half cup of cooked vegetables, fruit or juice, or one cup or one piece of raw fruit or vegetables.

Meat Group. Three servings per day of fish, poultry, eggs, or cheese provide protein as well as many vitamins and minerals. A serving is two ounces of meat, fish, or poultry; two eggs or two ounces of cheese; or one cup of dried beans, peas or nuts, or four tablespoons of peanut butter.

Grain Group. Four servings a day of grains and cereals supply a variety of vitamins, minerals, and some protein. A serving is one slice of bread or one cup of cereal or one-half cup of pasta, rice, or grits.

Milk Group. Two servings a day of milk or other products provide various vitamins and some protein. A serving is one cup of yogurt or milk, one and one-half ounces of cheese, one cup of pudding, one and three-quarter cups of ice cream, or two cups of cottage cheese. However, many doctors now minimize dairy use for AIDS patients.

Eating Problems

Lack of appetite (anorexia) is common among people with AIDS for many reasons, including depression, fatigue, nausea, and infection. Some approaches to dealing with lack of appetite include the following:

Altered Sense of Taste. Protein foods are a problem. Some people report that red meat in particular is either tasteless or metallic, like mush or sawdust. Try different seasonings or try using pickles or lemon juice on your meat. Eat poultry or fish instead. Since appetite is usually better in the morning, try to get at least one-third of the day's calorie and protein requirements into the breakfast meal. Eating the dinner meal at breakfast-time is one possibility. Use custards, eggnogs, or commercial liquid supplements between meals. Experiment with different temperatures for foods. High-protein foods eaten at room temperature or colder (ice cream, gelatin salads with cottage cheese, and fruit stuffed with nut butters) may have a more acceptable taste.

Depression. For most people, eating is a social event; thus the surroundings make a difference to the appetite. Share mealtimes with others when possible. An attractive table setting, flowers, a glass of wine, and music will go a long way toward making eating more enjoyable.

Fatigue. Many people are often too tired to cook or go out for food. Investing in a microwave oven can make food preparation much easier. And freezers can be stocked with high-protein main courses. Individuals may choose to cook favorite dishes when their energy level is up and then freeze the dishes for later use during more tiring times.

Getting Full Too Fast. This is a common problem that can be partially resolved by eating small servings more frequently, by chewing foods slowly and thoroughly, and by reducing fluid intake with meals. Make part of the liquid you drink with your meals as nourishing as the meal itself by using nutritional supplements (Sustacal, Ensure, etc.). The secret to meeting nutritional needs, in this case, is to get as many calories into as small a package as possible. Sauces, gravies, and nutritional supplements make this task much easier.

Nausea. The smell of cooking food may contribute to your desire to eat or it may cause nausea. In that case, have someone else cook instead. Eat uncooked foods such as cottage cheese or cold soups as an attractive alternative. Greasy or fried foods might be a problem and should be avoided. If nausea is a considerable problem, consult your doctor. Doctors may be able to prescribe anti-nausea medication which can be taken about thirty minutes before meals.

Diarrhea

This may be worsened by food intake, especially when caused by lactose (e.g. milk) intolerance, high fiber, or high fat diets. It may also be a side effect of a particular medical treatment or a direct result of some infection. Determine the cause of the diarrhea, if possible. Consult your physician about the cause.

Lactose Intolerance. Lactose is a milk sugar found primarily in milk and dairy products and added to many other foods. It requires an intestinal enzyme (lactase) to promote its digestion and absorption. When lactase is lacking, diarrhea, gas, or cramping may occur. Many adults lack this enzyme. Lactose production may be inhibited by intestinal infection, antibiotics, or other treatments. Persons with AIDS can determine whether lactose intolerance is contributing to diarrhea by observing the effects of eliminating dairy products and high lactose foods from their diet. High lactose foods include milk, ice cream, cheese (except natural cheese aged ninety days or more), instant coffee, cocoa, chocolate and most chocolate beverages, cream and desserts with custard or cream filling. Soybean formulas, such as those sold as infant formulas, can be used to substitute for dairy products in many cases.

High fiber diets increase bulk and stimulate intestinal movement; therefore, whole grains in bread or cereals, fresh fruits, and vegetables should be avoided to reduce fiber content when diarrhea is a problem. High fat diets, including fried or greasy foods and meats, may worsen diarrhea.

What Nutritional Supplements Can I Use to Increase My Calorie Intake?

There are many commercially prepared supplements available, all of which have their own special merits. Reading labels is particularly important when trying to decide which products best meet a person's unique needs. Some of the characteristics to consider include the following:

- Flavor—various flavors are available, from vanilla to black walnut. Unflavored types can be flavored with your own extracts.

- Milk substitutes—if problems with lactose intolerance exist, soy-based formulas may be good substitutes.

- Calories—the calorie concentration of supplements vary from brand to brand. Isocal HCN and Magnacal have the highest number of calories per serving while Isomil has the lowest.

- Taste—some products taste better "on the rocks" while others are better at room temperature. Taste varies from person to person, so it is better to personally sample them rather than relying on the reports of others.

- Powder supplements—they are often worth evaluating in terms of how they can be added to other foods to fortify protein and calorie content. One powder is worthy of note: polycose is a glucose polymer which is not very sweet, so it can be added to or sprinkled on most food items to increase calorie content. Polycose does not have any other nutritional value; but for adding calories, it is worth trying.

How Else Can I Add Calories and Protein to My Diet?

Some suggestions for adding calories include the following:

a) Fortify milk by adding one cup of nonfat dry milk to one quart homogenized or low-fat milk.

b) Add butter or margarine (45 calories per teaspoon) to everything imaginable.

c) Use mayonnaise (100 calories per tablespoon) as a salad dressing.

d) Spread peanut butter (90 calories per tablespoon) on fruit or bread.

e) Use sour cream (70 calories per tablespoon) or yogurt for a vegetable dip, sauce, and in gravies.

f) Put whipped cream (60 calories per tablespoon) on desserts and jello salads.

Exercise

Exercise is important for maintaining circulation, muscle mass, and for improving your sense of well-being. People who are able to get outdoors should undertake a regular schedule of walking. Lifting weights is useful for everyone, including those who spend great amounts of time in bed. It is important to remember that exercising just until the point of fatigue is helpful, but pushing much beyond that point may be detrimental. Do only what you can. Physicians and physical therapists may help determine how to exercise with the safest benefits.

Dental Care

The mouth, believe it or not, plays a critical role in the care and promotion of overall good health of persons with AIDS. Dental care—including teeth and gums—can improve a personal sense of well-being, prevent some opportunistic infections, and maintain the ability to eat properly. Caring for your teeth pays off; therefore, get regular checkups and early diagnosis and treatment when a problem arises. (Please keep in mind that when you visit your dentist or oral hygienist, the typically high amount of blood exposure requires that gloves and masks be worn and other precautions taken to reduce the risk of AIDS transmission. The Centers for Disease Control now advises dental care professionals to take these precautions with all patients.)

Prevention and Maintenance

Contact a dentist as soon as you are diagnosed with AIDS or ARC or HIV infection. Immediate care and regular checkups (as recommended by your dentist) can reduce your risk of many opportunistic infections. Use these routine oral hygiene guidelines:

- brush regularly (use a soft brush);
- get regular check ups;
- floss regularly;

- don't eat too many sweets, and rinse or brush soon after eating. If an infection or lesions are present in the mouth, you may find Toothettes (little sponge-tipped swabs) easier or gentler to use.

Treatment

An aching or diseased mouth can make life very uncomfortable. Eating is difficult, thus making proper nutritional intake problematic. And additional infections may be more likely to develop. All people with AIDS, ARC, or HIV infection should be careful to follow these guidelines:

a) Seek treatment early. Problems that continue may be more difficult to treat and, if neglected, may lead to complications.

b) If you need oral surgery or extensive work, your dentist may prescribe antibiotics to prevent opportunistic infections.

c) Information regarding infections and treatment should be shared between you and your dentist and your physician to ensure that:
   — prescribed drugs have no conflicting or interfering side effects;
   — your treatment plan is appropriate;
   — your overall condition allows for surgery (or other necessary work) at this time.

Dental care is often difficult to obtain for those with AIDS. If you are in need of these services, you might get a referral from your doctor or your local AIDS organization.

General Hygiene Measures and Risk Reduction

Stephen Strigle, B.S., C.T. (ASCP)
and Judith Spiegel, M.P.H. *

Good hygiene is important in daily living for two reasons. First, living in a clean environment generally makes people feel better and often makes friends and family more comfortable during their visits. Second, good hygiene is just plain healthy. There is no question that living in a clean environment and practicing good hygiene substantially reduces the risks of contracting many infections. At the same time, there is no reason why people with AIDS, ARC, and HIV infection who follow basic hygiene guidelines should not be able to share their homes with others. A few basic rules to follow are:

a) Keep living areas well-ventilated but at a comfortable temperature.

b) Keep all areas not just neat but clean.

c) Maintain personal cleanliness through daily bathing and dental hygiene. Most importantly, wash your hands after using toilet facilities, after contact with body fluids (blood, saliva, semen, urine, feces), and before eating or cooking.

---

*adapted from instructions by Helen Schietinger, R.N., and Grace Lusby, R.N.

In the Bathroom

Above all else, always wash your hands after using toilet facilities. There is no need for separate toilet facilities; however, it is important to keep them clean. Toilet seats and fixtures should be cleaned routinely with a 1:10 dilution of household bleach. A little full-strength bleach can be poured directly into the toilet bowl for disinfection.

Mop the bathroom floor at least weekly and clean up spills. Again, a 1:10 dilution of bleach (one part bleach to nine parts water) can be used to disinfect the floor and shower stalls. (Athlete's foot is caused by a fungus which bleach will kill.)

Use one sponge (or washrag) for dishes and eating areas, and another for cleaning up messes that might involve human waste or body fluids. It is wise to wear rubber gloves when cleaning bathroom areas or spills on the floor. For easier disposal, you might want to use plastic waste basket liners.

In the Kitchen

People with AIDS, ARC, and HIV infection can safely prepare food for others as long as hands are washed before beginning. (It is also a good idea not to lick your fingers while cooking or tasting.)

Certain foods are best avoided by people with AIDS. These include organically grown food (these may be fertilized with human or animal wastes). If these foods are used, they should be cooked. Organic lettuce, however, is not safe. Unpasteurized milk and milk products have been associated with salmonella infections in the past, and these infections are not well tolerated by people with AIDS.

There is no need for separate utensils or dishes, but all of these must be washed in *hot* soapy water. Use water as hot as possible (gloves might be needed); it might help to turn up the water heater. If necessary, put utensils in a stainless steel bowl and pour boiling water over them. Automatic dishwashers are especially helpful as the water gets very hot.

Do not use the same sponge or rag for dishes that is used to clean up floor spills. Remove all food from the vicinity of the sink when you dump water used for mopping up the floor.

Clean the inside of the refrigerator regularly with soap and water to control molds. Dispose of old, stale food from the refrigerator on a regular, timely basis.

Laundry

Clothing, bed linens, and towels should be washed in a washing machine using hot water and household bleach. (Use the dilutions on the product label.) Laundry can be dried in an automatic dryer on a hot setting or it can be drip-dried in sunlight. Clothing or bed linens that are soiled with fecal matter, urine, or semen should be washed separately.

Personal Hygiene

Bathing/Washing. People with AIDS should keep their bodies clean. Such care may reduce the number of infectious agents on the skin which are capable of causing opportunistic infections. Liquid soap dispensers are worth considering (and may be less harsh on the skin), and towels should *not* be shared. Perhaps the most important part of bathing or hand washing is rinsing well. This is the process which actually carries away the germs and dirt.

Cleansing Enemas and Douches. Use a one-time disposable unit whenever possible. Dispose of units with care, and never share equipment. Keep your personal kit clean by boiling the nozzle in hot water after each use. Though considered by some to be a hygienic practice, remember that too much cleansing may be harmful because it may irritate the mucous membranes of the rectum and/or the vagina. It may also wash away some of the valuable organisms that keep the system in balance.

Dental Hygiene. Even if teeth may be brushed regularly, the mouth is usually full of germs. A toothbrush should *never* be shared whether users are healthy or not. The gums are fragile and can bleed easily, providing a potential risk for others. Other teeth-cleaning devices such as toothpicks, dental floss, and water picks should never be shared. (There is no danger, however, in sharing the same dental floss dispenser.) After cleaning teeth or dentures, rinse water should be disposed of properly down the sink. Glasses used for rinsing should be washed with hot, soapy water.

Feminine Hygiene. Sanitary napkins and tampons can be infectious; these should be disposed of properly in a lined, protected waste container.

Nail Hygiene. Fingernails and toenails are usually dirty since dirt and organisms can easily lodge under them. Keep nails clean and away from the mouth.

Secretions. Despite findings that the AIDS virus can be isolated from saliva, epidemiological evidence argues against the transmission of AIDS via saliva or other respiratory secretions. Studies of people sharing households with others who have AIDS or ARC, or are infected with AIDS virus, have shown no spread of the virus as a result of casual contact among household members. Pneumocystis carinii pneumonia cannot be transmitted to persons with normal immune system function, but it could be transmitted between persons with AIDS. (However, other infectious agents can be transmitted between healthy and immune-suppressed individuals.) Therefore, individuals should be careful to cover their mouths and noses with a tissue when coughing or sneezing. Because of the potentially infectious nature of oral and nasal secretions, always dispose of tissues properly and wash hands immediately after exposure to secretions.

Shaving. Razors can harbor minute particles of blood and also irritate the skin. Therefore, razors should never be shared.

Pets and Their Care

First, persons with any type of immune deficiency must be cautioned against having pets. If such individuals now have or are considering acquiring a new pet, physicians should be consulted to determine whether any risks exist.

Those people who do have pets must be careful with their waste products and with their litter boxes. In fact, persons with AIDS should not directly clean animal spills, litter boxes, aquariums, or bird cages. Many opportunistic organisms are harbored in waste products.

Health needs of pets should be attended to, especially any vaccines or other shots. Pets that are exclusively indoor animals and isolated from other animals pose the least risk.

General Housecleaning Rules

Keep a positive, fun outlook on these activities. As much as cleaning may be disliked, living areas will most likely be more appreciated if they are kept clean.

Home Care

by Jennifer Lang, R.N., M.N.

Because of personal preferences and the difficulty of placing persons with AIDS in skilled nursing facilities, many patients with AIDS who are too sick to care for themselves are cared for in the home by professionals, friends, or family members. The following guidelines, along with the general hygiene measures in the previous section, should be helpful in providing home care.

Hygiene. In the person with fevers and night sweats, bathing becomes not only a hygienic necessity, but also a refreshing relief. For the person who has enough strength to get out of bed, but not enough to stand alone in the shower, placing a stool or chair in the shower stall or bathtub is helpful. The use of a shower-hose attachment to the faucet cuts down on spray considerably. Getting in and out of the bathtub may be difficult for someone with weak leg muscles; therefore, a chair in a shower stall is probably easier.

If unable to get out of bed, a daily bed bath can be accomplished with the use of a basin of lukewarm water, a face cloth, bath towel, and mild soap. Remove the bed covers, the patient's pajamas, and cover the patient with a sheet, large towel, or light blanket to prevent chilling. Wrap the face cloth around your hand to form a mitten and wash the face first. Avoid soap on the face since it is hard to remove if it gets in the eyes. Wash, rinse, and pat dry with the towel. Wash hands and arms next—first with soapy wash cloth, then rinse and wipe soap off, patting dry. Wash and dry each arm separately to avoid chilling. The front of the chest and neck comes next, followed by the abdomen, back, buttocks, and genitalia. Feet and legs go last. If the water gets too soapy, dirty, or cold, change with fresh water. Bath water should be lukewarm (104 degrees F). Wear rubber gloves while bathing the patient, particularly when washing the rectal or genital area. This is particularly important if there is any fecal soiling. The application of lotions, especially to feet and elbows, not only refreshes but also protects the skin from skin friction.

Oral Hygiene. Daily mouth care is very important. If thrush is present, more frequent care (every four hours) is required. If toothbrush bristles cause discomfort or bleeding, use a face cloth, or commercially available Toothettes (sponge-tipped swabs) to clean teeth and gums. Mouth rinses with warm salt water (one teaspoon per eight-ounce glass of water) are helpful. Hydrogen peroxide in a 50:50 dilution with warm water can also be used. If your patient cannot cooperate with mouth care, the mouth can be kept open by placing a wooden tongue depressor (blade vertical) between upper and lower teeth while cleaning is accomplished. The patient who cannot cooperate may also be confused and is capable of choking. In such a case, do *not* use mouth rinses.

Shaving. The use of an electric razor is recommended as the risk of bleeding increases with a regular blade razor. If a regular razor is used, the care-giver should wear disposable rubber gloves while shaving the patient.

Changing Bed Linens. Ideally, the patient will be strong enough to get out of bed while the bed linen is changed. If not, remove the top linen, have the patient turn on his side to one side of the bed, roll the dirty sheet like a sausage, and push it as far as possible under the patient's back. Fit the clean sheet onto the empty side of the bed and fold the loose (untucked) portion of the clean sheet in an accordian fashion close to the patient. Then, you can roll the patient onto the fresh sheet; remove the old linen; and lastly, tuck in the remaining portion of the clean sheet neatly under the mattress. Apply a clean top sheet and blankets, if needed. Bed linen that is not soiled does not need to be changed daily, but a fresh, unwrinkled bottom sheet does improve comfort. For the patient who has difficulty controlling urination or bowel movements, the use of disposable plastic lined underpads may protect linen and mattress from frequent soiling. These are commonly called "Chux" and can be purchased from drugstores or hospital equipment rental stores.

There are several advantages to using a rented hospital bed. The mattresses are covered and easily cleaned. Since most of them are electric, they can be raised to a high position while changing linens to protect the care-giver's back, and then lowered for the patient's safety. The head and knee sections can also be raised and lowered to vary comfort and feeding positions for the patient. When prescribed by a physician, most insurance plans will cover the expense.

Meeting Nature's Demands. Whenever possible, the patient should be encouraged to use the bathroom—if for no other reason than to provide some exercise and promote a sense of independence. If this is not possible, then a urinal or bedside commode is a possible substitute. A bedpan, although difficult to use and also uncomfortable, may be a necessity for the patient who is not able to get out of bed. The use of underpads will protect bed linen in this case. For the patient who is not able to control bladder function, a condom catheter (described in the supply section) will prevent bed-wetting.

Useful Supplies and Equipment for the Home Care of the AIDS Patient

Almost all of the items listed below can be purchased or rented from either a drugstore or a hospital equipment establishment. When prescribed by the physician, many insurance plans will cover the expenses.

1) Disposable latex or vinyl gloves. They don't need to be sterile. Most come in boxes of 50 for approximately $14.00.

2) Disposable plastic-backed underpads to protect sheets from fecal or urinary soiling. Known as Chux, they come in several sizes and quantities, the largest being most useful.

3) Disposable face masks.

4) Plastic urinal, reusable.

5) Bedpan or bedside commode. A commode is helpful for the patient who can get out of bed but is not strong enough to get to the bathroom.

6) A Texas catheter, also known as a condom catheter, is a rubber sleeve which slips over the penis. A drainage tube which goes to a collection bag is attached to one end of the condom. This is helpful for the patient who is having difficulty controlling urination.

7) Hospital beds are particularly helpful for the AIDS patient who is not very mobile, since the bed height can be raised to protect the care-giver's back or lowered for the patient's safety. In addition, the head of the bed can be raised to facilitate eating or breathing.

8) Wheelchair. A collapsible wheelchair with brakes and a footrest which will fit easily into a car is a useful addition, particularly for getting from hospital parking lots to clinics.

9) Walker. A four-legged aluminum frame, which the patient moves in front of him, is helpful for the patient who is still mobile but has problems maintaining balance.

Precautions for Care-Givers

1) Wash hands before and after direct contact with the patient.

2) Wear disposable rubber gloves when:
   — bathing or cleansing the rectal or genital area;
   — giving mouth care;
   — emptying a bedpan, commode, or urinal;
   — shaving with a safety razor;
   — giving injections;
   — cleaning up vomit, urine, or stool;
   — cleaning toilet fixtures.

3) Wear an apron that protects clothing from shoulders to knees whenever giving care which may place you at risk of being soiled from fecal material, vomit, or urine.

4) Wear a face mask only when coming in close contact (within three feet) of a patient who is coughing sputum into the air.

5) Dispose of soiled plastic or paper items in a plastic garbage bag.

6) Wash aprons in hot water with detergents and household bleach.

7) Dispose of urine, stool, and vomit in the toilet.

8) Clean commodes and toilet fixtures with any disinfectant. A 1:10 dilution of household bleach is cheapest and effective.

9) The toilet brush used to clean toilet bowls or commodes should soak in a diluted bleach solution between uses.

10) Needles and syringes used to withdraw blood or give injections in the home should be saved for disposal in a small used coffee can, lined with a plastic bag, and covered with a plastic top. When the coffee can is full, make sure the plastic bag is inside the can and then place the can in a 350-450 degree oven until the plastic syringes have melted. Allow the can to cool, remove from the oven, cover with plastic lid, and dipose of in the trash.

Symptom Management

PNEUMOCYSTIS CARINII PNEUMONIA (PCP)

What to Watch for:

a) Shortness of breath under circumstances which would not normally make you short of breath.

b) Dry cough.

c) Unexplained fevers higher than 101 degrees, for more than twenty-four hours.

What to Do:

a) Record your temperature with a thermometer every four hours.

b) Drink plenty of fluids.

c) Call your doctor if the symptoms become worse or fail to improve over one or two days.

What Information to Give Your Doctor or Nurse:

a) Duration or shortness of breath in days or weeks. Is it getting worse, better, or staying the same? What makes it worse? Better?

b) Duration of cough. Are you producing any phlegm (sputum)? If so, what color, how much, and when?

c) What has your temperature been for the past twenty-four hours? What have you done or taken for it? Have these measures helped?

What to Expect:

What your doctor decides to do will depend on how serious he thinks the problem is. He may choose to:

a) Wait for further developments and keep in touch with you by phone.

b) Order a chest X-ray.

If You Are Admitted to the Hospital, You Might Expect:

a) Further chest X-rays.

b) A bronchoscopy—insertion of a flexible tube into the bronchial tube to obtain a lung tissue biopsy for PCP. Besides an open lung biopsy, this is the only way to make a definite diagnosis of PCP.

c) Arterial blood gases—removal of a small amount of blood from an artery in the wrist or the groin in order to determine how well your blood is oxygenated.

If You Do Have PCP, You Can Expect:

a) To have oxygen administered through your nose if the blood gases indicate a low oxygen level, or if you are short of breath.

b) To receive one of two antibiotics—either trimethoprim sulfasoxazole, a sulfa drug; or pentamidine, a drug obtained from the CDC.

c) Frequent chest X-rays.

Your Responsibilities as a Patient Are:

a) Communicate fears, needs, and concerns to staff. They care about you and want to help so that they can best meet your needs.

b) Understand what is happening to you, what is planned, and what the treatment goals are.

c) Continue to take your medicine after discharge from the hospital. PCP has a high recurrence rate, therefore prevention is essential. Unfortunately, the sulfa drugs Bactrim and Septra have a high rate of reactions. If you develop a rash and/or fever while on either of these medications, call your doctor.

ORAL CANDIDA (THRUSH)

What to Watch for:

a) Soreness of mouth or tongue, a "burnt" feeling.

b) Pain or difficulty in swallowing.

c) Appearance of white patches on the tongue or back of the mouth which do not come off with a toothbrush.

What to Do:

a) Make an appointment to be seen by your doctor. Unless this problem entirely prevents you from eating, it is not an emergency and can wait a few days for treatment.

b) While waiting for an appointment, you can rinse your mouth with a warm salt water solution (about one teaspoon salt per eight-ounce glass) every two to three hours.

What to Expect:

If your doctor thinks that it is candida, you may get a prescription for either Mycostatin(R) suspension or Ketoconazole(R) tablets. It is essential that you take the medication as directed, or it will not work. Do not skip doses!

Your Responsibilities:

Consult your doctor if the problem has not resolved after two weeks of medication.

WEIGHT LOSS

What to Watch for:

Unexplained weight loss of more than ten pounds in a month and which cannot be regained. (In AIDS, weight loss commonly occurs without reason and despite good appetite.)

What to Do:

a) Weigh yourself without clothes or shoes no more than once a week, and keep a record. Weigh yourself at about the same time of day.

b) Keep a food intake diary to determine calorie intake whenever you think you are losing weight. (See the "Nutrition and Exercise" in this section for more information.)

c) Try to eat a diet well balanced in fats, proteins, and carbohydrates.

d) If you are losing weight, maintain intake at a minimum of twenty calories per pound or ideal body weight (see "Nutrition and Exercise" in this section for specifics on how to determine this). You can do this by using sauces, gravies, Sustacol, Ensure, Carnation Instant Breakfast, and other liquid nutrient products.

e) If three large meals a day are difficult, split your total daily intake into six smaller meals.

f) If you continue to lose weight, call your doctor.

What Information to Give:

a) How many pounds have you lost over what period of time?

b) Approximately how many calories do you consume each day?

What to Expect:

If your weight loss has been excessive (more than twenty pounds in one month), you may be admitted to the hospital for evaluation and perhaps intravenous feedings.

Your Responsibilities Include:

a) Eat, even when you are not hungry.

b) Explore new ways of meeting nutritional needs.

c) If you do not feel well enough to cook for yourself, and no one else is available, ask your local AIDS organization for assistance in making arrangements to get help.

DIARRHEA

AIDS patients are particularly prone to intestinal parasites such as amoeba, giardia, and cryptosporidia. There are treatments available for amoeba and giardia, but not for cryptosporidia. Diarrhea may also occur without an identifiable cause.

What to Watch For:

a) More than six loose stools per day.

b) Watery, mucoid, or bloody stools.

c) If stool is bloody, does blood come before, with, or after the bowel movement?

d) Approximate volume of bowel movements.

What to Do:

a) Call your doctor and describe your stools; a stool specimen for parasites or bacterial culture may be required. Get stool containers from a hospital laboratory. If your doctor is concerned about cryptosporidia, a special container containing a preservative can be obtained. Stool specimens are more easily obtained if plastic wrap is placed across the toilet bowl to prevent the stool from falling into the toilet water.

b) If stool cultures are negative, but diarrhea persists, try altering your diet—avoid dairy products, spices, coffee, alcohol, and foods high in fat. Drink liquids at room temperature. Avoid fresh fruits and juices high in acid.

What to Expect:

a) If stools contain amoeba or giardia, you may be given a prescription for Flagyl. Medication that is not completed is not effective; take the entire regimen as directed. Alcohol intake while taking Flagyl may cause an adverse reaction.

b) Drugs that delay transit time from food ingestion to elimination may be prescribed (i.e., Lomotil).

c) There is no known treatment which will eliminate cryptosporidia, but medications can be prescribed which reduce discomfort.

Your Responsibilities as a Patient:

a) Take medication as prescribed.

b) Do not drink alcohol while taking Flagyl.

c) Maintain fluid intake (non-caffeinated) to prevent dehydration. (Chipped ice or popsicles may be easier to tolerate if diarrhea persists.)

d) Report symptoms of weakness, dizziness, or excessive weight loss.

DEHYDRATION

This occurs when there is excessive loss of body water due to fevers, sweating, diarrhea, or decreased fluid intake.

What to Watch for:

a) Dryness of oral mucous membranes and tongue.

b) Skin on back of hand when pinched (into tent shape) does not return to its place quickly.

c) The passage of very little (less than one cup) or no concentrated urine over a twelve-hour period. (Concentrated urine is dark yellow in color.)

d) Inability to take in as much fluid as is being lost in diarrheal stools.

e) Confusion—difficulty in remembering where you are or behavior that is strange for you.

f) Dizziness when standing.

What to Do:

a) Control fevers as advised by your physician.

b) Increase fluid intake with water, juices, Gatorade, popsicles, ice, etc.

c) Measure the amount of urine passed.

d) Call your physician if you start feeling more confused; cannot increase your urine output to at least a quart every twelve hours even after increasing fluid intake; or are having difficulty taking in enough liquids.

What Information to Give:

a) Temperature for past twenty-four hours.

b) Approximate amount of fluids taken in for past forty-eight hours.

c) Approximate amount of urine passed in past twenty-four hours.

d) The presence and/or severity of diarrhea.

e) Your weight today and comparison to what it was a week ago.

What to Expect:

If your doctor does not think you can manage at home, he may admit you to the hospital to give intravenous fluids.

Your Responsibilities as a Patient:

a) Maintain a fluid intake which is at least a quart more than your combined urine and stool output.

b) Be alert for signs of dehydration.

c) Report any concerns to your physician.

FEVERS

Usually fevers are a sign of infection, but AIDS is often accompanied by nighttime fevers and sweats for which no cause can be found.

What to Watch for:

a) Temperatures greater than 101 degrees.

b) The time of day when they occur.

c) Night sweats which soak through bed clothes and sheets.

d) Other signs of infection (sore throat, headache, cough, etc.)

What to Do:

a) Record temperature every four hours (not more often) for two to three days, and look for a pattern.

b) Discuss findings with your doctor—call sooner if other symptoms coincide with fevers.

c) Drink plenty of fluids to replace the water you lose through sweating.

d) Ask your doctor whether he/she prefers aspirin or Tylenol, and the preferred method of taking the medication.

What to Expect:

a) If your doctor suspects an infection, he/she may want to evaluate with blood or urine cultures, X-rays, etc.

b) If no cause is found and the fevers are related to AIDS, you can expect them to recur episodically and last for several days at a time.

Your Responsibilities as a Patient:

a) Rest when you are tired.

b) Consult with your doctor as to the best approach to take when fevers occur.

c) Maintain fluid intake to compensate for fluid loss through night sweats and increased metabolism. Gatorade may be helpful for restoring electrolyte balance.

FATIGUE

This is a common symptom with AIDS that may interfere with your lifestyle, lasting either for an indefinite period or occurring in cycles.

Your Responsibilities as a Patient:

a) Consult with your physician if fatigue prevents you from working or caring for yourself; becomes significantly worse; or is associated with cough, shortness of breath, or a new fever.

b) Maintain an exercise program which does not cause excessive fatigue but helps maintain muscle mass.

c) Inquire about eligibility for disability (financial assistance) if fatigue prevents you from working.

CHANGES IN MOOD, PERSONALITY, BEHAVIOR, SPEECH, OR MEMORY

The opportunistic infections which affect the brain or central nervous system may develop slowly and are accompanied by subtle changes in personality or speech. Spouses, close friends, or lovers are often the first to recognize these.

What to Watch for:

a) Changes in the way you respond to situations; that is anger for no reason, suspicions of others' behavior, desire to be alone (if it is uncharacteristic of you), difficulty coping with things that are not normally a problem.

b) Difficulty understanding or forming words.

c) Difficulty with balance or ability to walk; new weakness of an arm, leg, hand, or foot.

d) Severe headaches or neck stiffness.

e) Changes in the way close associates react to you.

f) Difficulty remembering where you are or recalling important events.

What to Do:

a) Ask those who know you well if they have noticed any changes in your behavior.

b) Discuss any concerns with your physician.

c) Don't allow yourself to think that you are going crazy.

What to Expect:

If your physician thinks your concerns may be valid, he/she may:

a) Hospitalize you to evaluate for opportunistic infection.

b) Allow you to stay home while he/she evaluates your symptoms further.

c) Recommend that you have someone stay with you to help, if needed.

Managing the Side Effects of Treatment for Kaposi's Sarcoma

Jennifer Lang, R.N., M.N.

Management of many of the treatment side effects are similar to those already described in "Symptom Management."

Nausea may occur as a side effect of any of the treatment programs. It is usually transient, and generally lasting for a few hours after treatment. Nausea and vomiting as a result of chemotherapy respond better to preventive approaches. Once vomiting starts, it is difficult to stop until it runs its course. Avoiding food intake prior to therapy may help. Your physician and chemotherapy nurse will be able to help you find the best method of dealing with the problem; they can prescribe anti-nausea medications when indicated.

Diarrhea may occur following radiation to the abdomen or as a result of some chemotherapy treatments. Diarrhea associated with radiation is due to inflammation of the lining of the intestines; it may be controlled with a low-fiber, lactose-free diet (lactose is the sugar substance found in milk products). Diarrhea following chemotherapy will usually run its course over a few hours and requires no treatment unless it persists.

Medications may also slow down intestinal activity. Constipation may occur as a side effect of vincristine or vinblastine (two chemotherapy drugs); it often occurs several days after therapy. Usually those bouts can be prevented with a high-fiber diet and high liquid intake. If there has been no bowel movement for more than three days and abdominal cramping occurs, it is best to consult a physician.

Mouth sores occur when the uppermost layer of cells covering the mucous membranes are lost. This can happen several days after treatment with chemotherapy, or the drug interferon, and can continue until new cells grow, in approximately seven days. Rinsing the mouth frequently with warm salt water is very helpful. Use a soft toothbrush or Toothettes (a sponge-tipped stick) to clean teeth. A medication called viscous xylocaine can be prescribed to reduce mouth pain, but the results are temporary and of short duration.

Hair loss can occur as a result of chemotherapy treatments. Interferon can cause a thinning of hair, but it generally does not bring on a total loss. The severity of hair loss as a result of chemotherapy varies from drug to drug. With vinblastine, it may be minor. With adriamycin, it may be major. Hair fall-out usually begins seven to fourteen days following treatment, and some new growth may be evident just prior to the next treatment. Following completion of chemotherapy, hair will return completely but sometimes with a different color or texture. In recent years, a technique which involves cooling the scalp with ice packs—to reduce the amount of chemotherapy reaching the hair follicles—has been found to delay hair loss in some situations. Given the fact that Kaposi's sarcoma is a skin tumor, scalp cooling is not recommended.

Lowered blood counts occur as a result of the treatment's effect on the bone marrow. The bone marrow responsible for producing the majority of blood cells is found in the ribs, sternum (breast bone), hips, vertebral column (backbone), skull, and upper arms. Radiation therapy which involves any of these areas will affect blood counts. Some chemotherapy drugs have more of an effect on blood counts than others. Interferon may also have an effect. Chemotherapy affects blood counts by temporarily arresting the ability of the bone marrow to produce new blood cells. White blood cells and platelets are especially sensitive to this effect and usually reach their lowest level seven to fourteen days after treatment. Chemotherapy treatments are usually spaced apart to allow time for the bone marrow to recover prior to the next treatment. When counts are at their lowest level, patients are at risk, particularly for developing infections, bruising, or bleeding easily from cuts. The appearance of new symptoms of fever or easy bruising should alert chemotherapy patients to the possibility of low counts which need evaluation. Being in crowds and participating in activities that involve vigorous physical contact should be avoided at this time.

Fevers. Patients receiving the drugs bleomycin or interferon may experience fevers, chills, muscle aches, or pains within a few hours of treatment. These are expected side effects and can be minimized with medications such as Tylenol and antihistamines (for bleomycin) when indicated.

Numbness and Tingling of Fingers. These are temporary toxic side effects of vinblastine or vincristine and should be reported to a physician at the next appointment so that subsequent doses of chemotherapy can be reduced.

Impotence. Some chemotherapy agents (vincristine and vinblastine) may temporarily interfere with the ability to achieve an erection. This will resolve spontaneously following discontinuance of these drugs.

[Editor's note: A "Self-Care Data Flow Sheet is included in Appendix Three to help you and your care-givers to track symptoms and medications in an organized fashion.]

Section Seven

A Practical Perspective

The primary purpose for getting your affairs in order is to provide peace of mind for yourself and to ensure minimal difficulties for the significant people in your life...If you are confronted with a life-threatening illness, do you need to worry as well about how your spouse, parents, family, friends, or lover will ever find or sort through your personal and financial records?

"Taking Care of Business"

Taking Care of Business

Durable Power of Attorney for Health Care

Tapping Social Services

Benefits Counseling

Understanding Your Insurance Policies

Taking Care of Business

More often than not, most of us overlook the details of preparing for our future—whether near or distant. When a problem or crisis arises, we often are poorly equipped to respond. The purpose of this chapter is to provide a basic framework and resources with which to handle the future. You may never have need for many of these services, but it is best to be prepared just in case. You will probably also find that it is easier to deal with legal matters while healthy and calm rather than when you face illness, stress, or time limitations.

This time can be an opportunity to think about your current needs and those that might develop. Certainly each person's needs are different. You may have experienced job or housing discrimination as a result of an AIDS or ARC diagnosis. If you believe this to be the case, you may wish to discuss the situation with staff members from your local AIDS organization or with a legal counselor. A few communities around the country—and several in California—have outlawed any AIDS-related discrimination. As a result, you may have the power of the law behind your complaint. Contact your local human rights commission if one exists, the county legal aid society, or your private attorney for more information and help. Several individuals have challenged successfully what they thought was discrimination by employers, landlords, and insurance companies. (See Appendices in Section Ten for a list of organizations that may help you with these concerns.)

Other legal issues to consider include estate planning, durable power of attorney for health-care decisions (a mechanism for assigning decision-making authority to a competent person of your choice), wills, and funeral arrangements. Some of these matters involve time limits after which they either become effective or outdated. It is important to consider these and plan ahead. The following discussion provides a brief explanation of these issues. For more clarification, consult a legal counsel or an AIDS organization.

Will

Each person has estate problems that are unique for that individual. It is important to consider not only the disposition of one's estate after death, but also the tax consequences of such dispositions. It is necessary to review the manner in which your assets, that is, money and possessions are held and to make informed judgments concerning the advisability of changing the form of ownership during life. The benefits of life insurance, retirement plans, and IRA accounts should be coordinated with other aspects of the estate plan. Sometimes it is possible to arrange one's affairs during life so that there is no need for probate proceedings after death. These determinations require a careful look at all the facts involved. A person planning his or her estate status can greatly benefit from the help of an attorney trained in this process. References to probate and estate planning attorneys can be obtained through local Bar Association referral services; volunteer organizations also make referrals to qualified attorneys who provide their services on a total or partial volunteer basis. Many AIDS organizations provide such volunteer services.

Information Collection

The primary purpose for getting your affairs in order is to provide peace of mind for yourself, knowing that unforeseen developments will not totally disrupt your life, and to ensure minimal difficulties for the significant people in your life. Having basic financial and other information assembled in one place can greatly help you achieve this goal. Furthermore, collecting the proper information about your finances and resources is a critical part of estate planning with your attorney. (The information collection form developed by the San Francisco AIDS Foundation with the cooperation of the Bay Area Lawyers for Individual Freedom can be a helpful way to get your affairs in order. It is included at the end of this article.)

The following is a list of some of the materials you may need to provide to an attorney:

1) copies of deeds to real property;

2) copies of securities;

3) copies of notes showing debts to or owed by the person desiring a will;

4) copies of ownership certificates of automobiles, boats, etc;

5) copies of life insurance policies or certificates, retirement plans, IRA accounts, and their beneficiary statements;

6) copies of documents showing the exact manner in which bank and savings and loan accounts are held;

7) an estimate of the total value of the estate and of the total amount of obligations;

8) information concerning one's preference for funeral and burial arrangements;

9) copies of prior wills.

While it is true that a will properly signed may be upheld even if it is signed just before death, the least satisfactory way to develop an estate plan is to wait until the last minute. There are not only emotional reasons for taking care of these matters well in advance, but there are also legal reasons—such as whether or not undue influence was exerted over the person making the will, and whether or not the person had the mental capacity required by law to make these decisions. If you want to ensure that your wishes and plans are followed, consult a knowledgeable attorney. A social worker or your local AIDS organization can help you determine which services might be most helpful to you. These are issues which we should all consider.

[Editor's Note: "Getting Your Affairs in Order," a series of financial resources worksheets, is included in Appendix Three.]

Durable Power of Attorney for Health Care

Bernard Lo, M.D.

Despite continuing research, AIDS is still a fatal illness; patients and physicians face dilemmas about the use of life-sustaining treatment. Often by the time such decisions must be made, patients have become mentally incompetent to participate in the process. According to ethical and legal recommendations, decisions for incompetent patients should follow preferences they expressed while still competent.

Most AIDS patients have thought about life-sustaining treatment and about what treatments they would accept or decline. Too often physicians hesitate to discuss such matters for fear of upsetting the patient. In fact, patients are usually appreciative of the opportunity to do so. An open-ended question may be helpful in raising the issue, such as "Have you thought about how you want us to make decisions in case you become too sick to talk with us directly?"

Many people with AIDS want their partners or friends, rather than their biological families, to make judgments if they are unable to do so themselves. However, such partners have no legal standing to make decisions, and traditionally physicians turn to families to decide for incompetent patients.

Reprinted with permission from *AIDSFILE*, April 1986, Volume 1, Number 2.

Under California law, competent patients can ensure that their preferences will be carried out by a person of their choice if they execute a *Durable Power of Attorney for Health Care*. By completing this standard form, available from the California Medical Association, patients can appoint a proxy to make decisions in case they become incompetent. The proxy must follow the previously expressed wishes of the patient. If these are unknown or unclear, the proxy must act in the best interest of the patient.

It is advisable for the patient to give specific directives for care in likely situations. Some AIDS patients, for example, will not want intensive care of mechanical intubation (placing a tube, say, into the larynx to keep the air passage open) for treatment of pneumocystis carinii pneumonia or other severe infections. Others may desire experimental or innovative therapies even in severe illness.

The Durable Power of Attorney for Health Care form can be completed without assistance from a lawyer, but it must be notarized or witnessed. It allows the patient to check agreement with one of three statements of preference about care. These standard statements, however, are vague and ambiguous; it is better if patients express their preferences in more specific terms, by attaching an additional sheet. If physicians follow proxy directions in good faith, the law provides them immunity from civil malpractice suits, criminal charges, and professional disciplinary action. "The Durable Power of Attorney" is more comprehensive and flexible than the "living will" or "directive to physicians," which apply to terminal illness and are biased toward limiting treatment.

Although most AIDS patients have thought about life-sustaining treatment if they should become incompetent, few have completed a Durable Power of Attorney for Health Care. Providers of care need to educate their patients about this document and the protection and peace of mind it can afford. Through discussions with patients, physicians can ensure that patients' preferences are informed and specific, and reassure them that symptomatic treatment and emotional support will always be available.

Copies of the form are available through the California Medical Association, or by writing to Sutter Publications, P.O. Box 7690, San Francisco, CA 94120-7690 or call (415) 863-5522. The forms come with an explanatory pamphlet; one version is geared to physicians ("What Physicians Should Know about Durable Power of Attorney for Health Care") and one is for patients ("Your Health Care: Who Will Decide When You Can't?"). Single copies are $1.50. Large orders are priced at reduced rates. Enclose a remittance with your order and specify which pamphlet you would like (you may request some of each). Residents of other states should consult their local AIDS organization, county medical association, or their attorney to determine whether Durable Power of Attorney is a legal option in their state.

Tapping Social Services

Coleen Johnson, M.S.W., L.C.S.W.

Many persons with AIDS and ARC face the challenge of applying for social services. The experience can be smooth and gratifying or frustrating and unproductive. While some parts of applying are essentially "out of your hands," you can have a considerable effect on most of the application process. Keeping a positive, persistent attitude during the course of your applications is extremely helpful. Enlisting the help of sympathetic individuals is beneficial as well. Other ways to make things run smoothly are to maintain a polite but firm attitude with agency staffs, complete paperwork conscientiously, and prepare your application so as to reflect a convincing picture of someone who needs aid. If after all your diligent efforts you do not receive what you believe you are entitled to, there are ways to address your grievances effectively.

Many persons with AIDS learn of their diagnosis in the hospital, while others learn of it as an out-patient. Often one's first reaction is disbelief. Other feelings may include despair, anger, and sadness. It is difficult to begin work toward any goals when your feelings are so fresh and confusing. Take some time to allow yourself to process what is happening before you make any major decisions such as whether to apply for social services.

One very important piece of information that you will need to obtain from your physician is whether or not you have AIDS according to the Centers for Disease Control (CDC) definition. Occasionally, a physician may be reluctant to give out this information. *Be insistent* that he or she provide you with this as soon as possible so that you can begin to make decisions about your future. Your physician will need to make certain tests to establish a diagnosis of AIDS, but should inform you of the results soon after he or she knows them. This is important because if one has CDC defined AIDS, it is much easier to establish eligibility for social services.

Another important point to consider is whether the decisive factor in your diagnosis is a positive biopsy for Kaposi's sarcoma (KS) or an opportunistic infection such as a bronchoscopy-proven case of pneumocystis carinii pneumonia (PCP). Some individuals have both the opportunistic cancer and opportunistic infections. There is some indication that those individuals who contract only KS may be the most able to continue in their jobs. It is important to discuss with your physician what he or she expects regarding the course of your illness. Ask him or her to be as realistic and honest as possible, and explain that you will be making important decisions based on the information he or she gives you. You may want to take the physician's personal style into account here: Has he or she always downplayed the seriousness of your physical condition, or has he or she been gravely concerned about every lab test? This may give you an idea of how to interpret what your physician tells you about returning to work.

If you are in the hospital and are having difficulty coming to a decision about returning to work or dealing with your feelings about your diagnosis, you can request a psychiatric consultation or visit with a hospital social worker. In most metropolitan areas there are local AIDS-related organizations that can send someone to visit with you and discuss these matters. The advantage of doing this while you are still in the hospital is that the social worker can help you with the applications process. Ideally, the social worker should come to visit and assess your needs without your asking, but in reality you may have to ask for one. Be insistent that a social worker comes to see you if there should be a delay of more than one day. Remember, after you are discharged you will no longer have access to this helpful person.

The social worker or psychiatric consultant should be able to help you talk about your feelings toward applying for public assistance. You may feel too proud to apply, thinking that you've always paid your way so far, so why stop now? Or the word "disability" may be offensive to you, bringing up feelings of helplessness. These feelings may cause you to delay your applications, which can be problematic three months down the line if your savings give out and you aren't well enough to return to work. One good reason *not* to apply is that you are definitely returning to work with your physician's support or have a private disability plan. In any event, as always, it is better to be safe than sorry. You run far less risk by applying early and having to cancel applications than by not applying and then finding that you are unable to return to work.

In the long run, the decision about returning to work or applying for social services is yours. Some persons with AIDS feel more comfortable continuing with their regular schedule, in order not to think about their illness all the time. Others prefer to remove any source of stress from their lives and rest as much as possible.

Applying for social services can be trying. One of the best things you can do is enlist the help of others. Besides the hospital social worker or representative from a local AIDS-related agency, you may want to ask a friend or family member to help you through the process. Choose someone who is confident and whom you trust. Ask them to accompany you to various agencies, or to intervene on your behalf when you are too ill or frustrated to do so. Do everything you can on your own. It will help you to feel more independent, and then your friends and family will be happy to help when you really need them.

Another important thing to do is to begin a notebook. Note all pertinent information concerning your application. Entries might look like this:

Date: May 15, 1987
Time: 1:30 p.m.
Contact: Coleen Johnson
AIDS Project L.A.
Phone: (213) 876-8951

Subjects Discussed: *Ms. Johnson recommended that I apply for both California State Disability Insurance (SDI), Federal Disability (SSD) and Supplemental Security Income (SSI). I applied for these upon leaving the hospital. Set* *up an appointment with her to discuss this in detail May 19, 1987, at 3 p.m., AIDS Project offices, 3650 Wilshire Blvd., Ste. 300.*

Date: May 19, 1987
Time: 3:00 p.m.
Contact: Coleen Johnson
Phone: (213) 876-8951

Subjects Discussed: Ms. Johnson suggested that I apply for Medi-Cal in addition to what I have already done. Gave me the address and contact person, Mr. Jones at (213) 123-7654.

Date: May 26, 1987
Time: 8:30 p.m.
Contact: Ms. Smith, Eligibility Worker, Department of Social Services
(Mr. Jones was out sick)
Phone: (213) 123-7654

Subjects Discussed: Ms. Smith stated I was ineligible for Medi-Cal.

Date: May 26, 1987
Time: 9:00 a.m.
Contact: Coleen Johnson
Phone: (213) 876-8951

Subjects Discussed: Am I ineligible for Medi-Cal? Coleen says no. She'll call Ms. Smith and her supervisor.

Date: May 26, 1987
Time: 1:30 p.m.
Contact: Coleen Johnson
Phone: (213) 876-8951

Subjects Discussed: Coleen says she yelled at Ms. Smith and her supervisor, Ms. McDonald (321-1237). I should go back tomorrow at 8. Don't be discouraged. Call her if any other problems.

Date: May 30, 1987
Time: 1:30 p.m.
Contact: Coleen Johnson
AIDS Project L.A.
Phone: (213) 876-8951

Subjects Discussed: Ms. Smith very apologetic and helpful. Completed paper-work, should hear within three months.

If you do this, it will save you a lot of trouble. It will also enable you to follow up on people who gave you false information, were rude, or "AIDS phobic." Do not hesitate to ask in a polite manner for the name of someone's supervisor if there is a problem. Advise the supervisor of the problem and ask for their help. Usually having an agency helping you (such as a local AIDS Project) will get much quicker results. Do not be afraid to use the names of personal political contacts or other powerful persons. Many public or govern-ment assistance agencies have a person responsible for AIDS clients. You may wish to inquire about this.

When filling out applications, do not attempt to complete all the paper-work in one day. This can be mentally and physically fatiguing. Instead, set aside several periods when you can work on this over a week or two. An impor-tant point to remember is that public assistance is for people who are poor and disabled. If you are independently wealthy and actually able to work as well as before, the government is not going to be interested in giving you money. If you have stocks and savings accounts, you are expected to use most of these assets for your expenses before applying for financial aid. There is some examination of your finances retroactive to your application, so do not attempt to hide your assets by putting them in your friend's or parent's name the day before you apply.

It is important to include *all* details in reference to your physical status. Include all symptoms (memory loss, lack of energy, weight loss, chronic diar-rhea, poor concentration, etc.) with pertinent dates, physicians seen, and hospitalizations. In order to be eligible for most assistance, you must be con-sidered "permanently disabled" for a projective period of one year. This means that you are completely unable to work in *any* type of function. So you must convince the funding agency of this with the help of your physician(s).

There are exceptions to every rule. Programs differ from state to state. Some may allow shorter periods of disability or larger bank accounts. If you are not hospitalized and need assistance through the application process, a psy-chiatric social worker at your local community mental health center may be able to help you to sort out the different programs available to you, and your feelings as well.

What is fairly consistent from state to state are the Social Security pro-grams. One is Social Security Disability (SSD). This pays a certain amount per month for disabled persons, provided you have paid into it (i.e., it was withheld from payroll checks). Another program, Supplemental Security Income (SSI), brings your income up to a base level either with SSD or separate from it. The Social Security office closest to you can be found by looking in the phone book under U.S. Government. Other pertinent agencies can be located in the same manner under State and Local Government listings. Leaf through these pages of your phone book to familiarize yourself with any potentially helpful programs. Some cities have information and referral services which may help you find less obvious programs to assist you.

If you do not get results from your application that you believe to be fair, inquire about the redress of grievances. Follow through on the process with the same methods you used for your initial applications. Remember to keep a positive, persistent attitude, use others for support, and be assertive. Also remember that many other persons with AIDS have done what you are attempting and have succeeded. Good luck.

Benefits Counseling

Tristano Palermino

People with AIDS and AIDS-related complex (ARC) are coping with the realities common to others having a life threatening illness. Being ill and often unable to remain employed, they must depend on disability programs for financial support. Unfortunately, most people will be forced to live on 40 to 60 percent of the income they earned while employed. Most people receive less than $800 per month and may receive between $367 per month and $533 per month. Most people do not know what disability programs are available to them until they become disabled, and getting accurate information then can be difficult.

People who are employed fear that making inquiries about benefits status may arouse the suspicions of employers with regard to their health and suitability for work. I counseled a twenty-six-year-old man with Kaposi's sarcoma who paid $3,400 in cash to medical providers rather than use his group insurance plan for fear his employer would learn he had AIDS. He would not contact the personnel department of his company for disability information for fear his supervisor would hear he had done so. In California, employers are required to provide benefits information once during the course of a person's employment. It is usually provided at the time of hiring. Many people with AIDS and ARC experience difficulty in obtaining accurate, straightforward information about disability income and medical coverage. Many people with AIDS have resigned from jobs in order not to disclose their disease. This is unfortunate since some may lose disability benefits because some disability programs, such as the California State Disability Insurance program, pay only if one becomes disabled while working; one cannot quit a job and apply for SDI benefits later.

There are many disability programs, all with varying eligibility requirements (an explanation of all California disability programs appears at the end of this article). An employer may offer a private disability plan, may participate in the California State Disability Insurance program, may do both or neither. For persons who have been determined disabled for more than one year, Social Security disability benefits begin five months subsequent to the time they are deemed "disabled." Persons with sporadic or broken employment records, or self-employed persons who have not paid into Social Security or the state disability program, may be ineligible for all disability programs, except Supplemental Security Income (SSI) through the Social Security Administration, or General Assistance Disability (GA), the county program for indigent disabled persons in San Francisco, which pays $228 monthly plus food stamps ($79).

A person's response to receiving disability benefits will vary based on his or her readiness to accept being identified as "disabled," whether or not income benefits will be perceived as sufficient to live on, and on his or her experience with the benefit process. For some, benefit awards will be a welcome relief. Many people with ARC, for example, have difficulty "proving" they are in fact disabled by Social Security criteria and therefore live on County Public Assistance, which is considerably less.

For some it represents the "beginning of the end." No longer being able to work raises questions, such as, Will I ever return to work? Am I going to get even sicker? Feelings of anger, rage, and hopelessness may be exacerbated by inadequate benefit awards, bureaucratic procedures, and insensitive or homophobic claims representatives.

Although AIDS affects all age groups, the majority of people with it at this time are twenty to fifty years of age. Most have never had a serious illness before. Asking for help may be difficult. Many have never had contact with social service and public assistance programs. Application procedures may require personal information which the client feels is "none of their business."

Fear of AIDS or homophobia on the part of benefit representatives can further distress the client, who is already concerned about confidentiality: Who will learn of my diagnosis? Who has access to information? Many people with AIDS have lost their apartments, roommates, family support, or careers after other people have disclosed their diagnosis.

Social Security Administration Programs: SSI and SSA

There are two programs for the disabled that are administered by the Social Security Administration:

1) Supplemental Security Income (known as SSI); and
2) Social Security Disability (known as Social Security or SSA).

These programs have two main criteria that determine eligibility. For SSI, medical condition and current financial situation (monthly income, assets, etc.) are assessed. For SSA, medical condition is assessed, and employment history is reviewed to see how much and how long the claimant has paid into Social Security (FICA on wage stub) through employers.

Both SSI and SSA use the same medical criteria to determine disability. "Disability" is defined as any medical condition (physical or mental) which prevents or is expected to prevent one from working for a minimum of twelve months. People who have a Centers for Disease Control (CDC) diagnosis of AIDS (KS, PCP, etc.) are automatically presumed disabled, thereby meeting the medical criteria for both SSI and SSA. People who have an AIDS-related diagnosis are evaluated on a case-by-case basis, but are not automatically presumed disabled.

In order to qualify for SSA benefits, one must be determined disabled and must have paid into the Social Security system through employers five of the last ten years. This means one must have worked in a job or jobs where Social Security taxes (FICA) were withheld from the paycheck. SSA benefits are payable no earlier than five months after onset of disability. There is no fixed amount that is paid. The amount of benefits depends entirely on earnings: how much and how long one has paid into the Social Security system.

In order to qualify for SSI, one must be disabled and have a financial need. If one is disabled and has no income, or less than $524 per month, one is eligible for SSI. One does not have to have worked to receive SSI benefits.

Basic Eligibility Criteria Are:

1) Assets cannot exceed $1,600;
2) Monthly income must be below $524; and
3) If one owns a house, one must live in it to be eligible for SSI.

The general processing time for an SSI application is between one and three months. Benefits are retroactive to the date that one applied for them. SSI benefits pay up to $504 per month if one has no other income. If one gets $250 a month from state disability, for instance, then SSI will pay $504 less $250, which is $254 per month. One may be eligible for up to $527 per month if part of one's benefits is from Social Security Disability.

State Disability Insurance Program (SDI)

The California State Disability Insurance Program is administered by the State of California Employment Development Department.

Eligibility Is Limited to:

1) Persons who are employed by an organization which participates in the program (refer to your pay stubs, section SDI);

2) Persons who are self-employed and have elected to participate in the SDI program;

3) Individuals who receive unemployment or Worker's Compensation. They cannot, however, receive SDI and unemployment concurrently.

To qualify for benefits, one must be currently participating in the program at the time of disability. "Disability" includes any illness or injury, either physical or mental, that prevents the applicant from doing his or her regular or customary work. The amount of benefit payment, ranging from $50 to $224 per week, depends on wages received and SDI premiums paid during a twelve-month base period. Benefits are payable retroactively to the date the disability began to affect one's work, and benefits usually last one year.

General Assistance (GA)

General Assistance is administered by the City and County of San Francisco and provides basic emergency room and board. Eligible clients receive $144 twice per month, totaling $288 monthly. To receive benefits the net monthly income added to non-exempt personal property must be less than the *maximum GA grant amount*, which for one person is $288 per month.

Food Stamps

The Food Stamp program is a federally funded, county-administered program designed to assist people with low incomes in order to supplement their dietary needs. The monthly allotment of food stamps varies depending on the amount of income. A person who receives General Assistance is allowed $79 a month in food stamps. The amount of food stamp allotment decreases with any increase of income above that level. SSI recipients are not eligible for food stamps.

Medi-Cal

Medi-Cal is the state of California's equivalent to the federally mandated Medicaid program. The general medical and financial criteria for eligibility are very similar to the SSI requirements (see SSI). If one is eligible for SSI, one is automatically eligible for Medi-Cal and, therefore, does not need to apply for Medi-Cal separately. People who have a CDC defined AIDS diagnosis are presumed disabled for the purposes of Medi-Cal. If one has monthly income or assets over the Medi-Cal cutoff point, one may still be eligible if one pays a share of cost per month.

Understanding Your Insurance Policies

Brent O. Nance, CLU, RHU

This article is primarily written for persons with AIDS/ARC who have concerns about their insurance policies, including health, life, and disability. Two other groups will find this information helpful: people caring for persons with AIDS/ARC and those who are concerned about their own insurance needs. Even under the best circumstances, reading and understanding your insurance policies is a bit like learning a foreign language. However, with this guide (and a little patience and effort) you will have a greater understanding of your coverages, and know what they will do for you and what to expect. This understanding will help you to get the most from your benefits and make the handling of your paperwork easier. It should also help reduce your stress level by knowing the what, when, and how of your coverages.

If you do not have a copy of your group insurance plan, contact your employer to obtain one. If you're covered under individual plans, contact your insurance carriers for a duplicate copy.

I. YOUR INSURANCE AND CONTRACTUAL RIGHTS

Keeping Records

I cannot overemphasize the importance of keeping good records of your insurance papers, claims, and all communications with your insurance company. Don't throw out anything. You should keep a separate file for each type of policy you may have (health, disability, life). You may find it necessary to refer to the letters, bills, and claims information from time to time. It might be useful to start an insurance diary, and each time you talk to anyone regarding your policies you should jot down whom you spoke to, what was said, the date and time.

[Editor's note: Two valuable worksheets, "Summary of Your Health Coverage" and "Tracking Your Health Insurance Claims," are included in Appendix Three to help you organize your insurance information.]

Always have your insurance policy number, Social Security number, and all certificate numbers handy when you call your insurance company. Always use these numbers whenever you write to your new company. They must be able to identify who you are and what policy you are writing about. Some companies will issue you a claims number when you file for benefits. You will have to give this number to them any time you inquire about your claims. There is a sample form in this section you can use to record important information about your policy. This form can be copied and handed over to your doctors, hospital, or other health professionals as necessary.

Potential Problems: Pre-existing Conditions, Delays, Terminations of Coverage, and Exclusions

The best way to handle insurance problems is to avoid them in the first place. By fully understanding your benefits and contractual rights, you will be able to avoid problems and will know how to handle those that occur. The best time to learn about your coverage is before a claim occurs, or better yet, when you are shopping for proper protection. If you anticipate any type of insurance claim, then you should start this process now. Maybe you can appoint someone to help you understand and help with your insurance problems.

A great deal of stress and fear occurs when filling out HIV-related insurance claims: Will my insurance claims be paid? Can I be cancelled? What about pre-existing conditions, limitations. . . ?

It will help to explain general concepts first, many of which apply equally to health, disability, and life insurance. Insurance benefits can be denied for several general reasons including pre-existing condition limitations, policy exclusions, and claims occurring during the contestable period. If you have had coverage for more than two or three years, you generally will have few major problems. However, your benefits can be reduced or denied because you didn't follow guidelines on preauthorizations, reviews, exclusions, and limitations, or because you selected a health-care provider outside of your coverage plan's "approved list."

Most individuals and group contracts include a pre-existing condition clause. A pre-existing condition is an illness or condition which existed and was treated, or which should have been treated, before coverage started. This generally includes conditions for which you have seen a physician, taken medication, and had diagnostic tests for which prior symptoms existed. Pre-existing conditions are excluded from coverage for a specified period of time, generally six months to two years. Read your policy. After the stated time period full policy benefits will be honored. In some states a condition must first be diagnosed before it can be called pre-existing. Seek professional advice if necessary.

Knowledge of a positive HIV antibody or antigen (virus) may be considered evidence of a pre-existing condition. Other tests, such as monitoring T-cell counts, may also affect your insurability. In states where insurance companies are prohibited from obtaining these test results, *never discuss test results with an insurance company and be careful in any discussions with medical care providers about such results*. This advice is especially true for healthy individuals applying for insurance coverage. Discuss such information only "off the record" when talking to your health-care providers. *If you decide to take the AIDS antibody test, be sure your insurance program is in order first.*

Your policy may have been issued with a special exclusion rider for a medical or physical condition that existed before you applied for the policy. Medical insurance policies contain a long list of excluded conditions, treatments and other limitations. It is important to read and understand any exclusions contained in your contract.

Individual policies and some group policies contain contestable clauses. A policy can generally be contested (cancelled retroactively) for the first two/three years for material mis-statements of information on your application for coverage. If the insurance carrier can prove gross mis-statements of information on your application, claims may be denied and the policy may be cancelled with all premiums refunded. It is important to note that histories of sexually transmitted diseases, recreational drug use, unreported medical histories, and diagnostic tests have been enough to trigger cancellation of coverage. If this worries you, seek professional advice from an insurance counselor or attorney.

Be extremely careful in answering questions about sexual histories and illicit drug use. This information becomes part of your medical history and therefore is available to your insurance company. Any such adverse history may place your insurance coverage in jeopardy, especially if the coverage is considered contestable.

Once in a while, individuals denied benefits entitled to them face unreasonable delays, or have to deal with a claims examiner who refuses to treat them with the respect deserved. What can you do if this happens to you? First, write to the manager or vice president in charge of the claims department (an address can be found in your policy). List your complaints, giving all the necessary back-up information you kept (time and day of your calls, whom you spoke to, what was said, copies of letters, etc.). Most companies want to resolve your problem, if they can do so within the legal constraints of the policy.

If you feel that the insurance company is not living up to its contract, then you have several choices. You can write letters to the insurance company asking for reviews. If the review is negative, you can ask for outside peer reviews. This review is handled by professionals from both the Medical Associations and the insurance industry. Contact your local Medical Association office for information. You can also make a formal complaint, in writing, to the state Department of Insurance. Insurance companies have also been known to respond very well to threats of legal action appearing on a lawyer's letterhead.

Before filing formal complaints with the state Department of Insurance, or seeking an attorney, you should seek help from your insurance agent or the insurance office from which the policy was purchased. Sometimes a call to the insurance company from someone who can understand the jargon will help get the checks rolling. If not, the agent may be able to help explain where the paperwork is and what needs to be done to push it through the system. Local AIDS organizations may also offer insurance counseling services.

If benefits are denied or cancelled, you can question the insurance company's claims office, get insurance counseling through your local AIDS organization, and/or ask your own agent/broker to help you with any problems or questions you might have. Remember, it is the *duty* of the insurance company to inform you of your benefits. They work for you, so don't be shy about asking for details.

Keeping Your Coverages: Conserving Benefits with Continuation, Extensions, Conversions, and COBRA

Most people are covered by health insurance provided through their employer. Group benefits may include life, dental, vision, and disability income insurance. Group insurance generally provides excellent coverage while you are working. However, when your employment ends, your group benefits may end, change, or remain in effect. If you terminate employment, read your group insurance handbooks to determine if or how and under what conditions you can maintain your insurance benefits. You will usually find this information under sections titled: When Your Benefits Terminate, Disability Extensions, Conversion of Benefits, and Continuation of Coverage. More detailed information may usually be obtained from your carrier or your employer. However, a few general rules apply.

As of July 1, 1986, under a new federal law called COBRA, all employers of twenty or more employees who offer group plans must begin offering up to eighteen months of continuous insurance coverage for all terminating employees. Families of deceased employees may qualify for thirty-six months of continuous coverage. By June 30, 1987, all such plans must follow COBRA (with the exception of negotiated union plans that must conform when new contracts are approved). The provision includes medical, dental, vision, HMO plans, self-funded plans, public and private employers—excepting federal employer plans.

Under COBRA you can *buy* the same coverage by paying a monthly premium equal to 102 percent of monthly premium being charged to your employer. Employers must inform you of your COBRA rights within fifteen days of termination of your coverage; you will then have sixty days to exercise your rights. There are strong legal penalties imposed against employers who fail to comply. After the end of the eighteen months you can still exercise your conversion, and perhaps disability extensions. For smaller group plans and for those who might leave employment before your plan conforms to COBRA, other options generally apply.

If you have recently (in the last thirty-one days) left employment, and the continuation clause is not available, contact your former employer and get the necessary information about your rights to extend or convert your benefits.

Most group insurance plans offer the ability to extend and/or convert your group health and life benefits. The conversion rights in your group policy allow you to apply for an individual policy without answering health questions. The conversion policy may not offer the same level of benefits you had while employed and may be very expensive. However, these conversion rights, *if they are not exercised within the thirty-one days, will lose you forever your rights to convert your health insurance.*

If you are disabled *and* lose your employment, you may be able to have your group health and life coverages "extended" under a disability extension clause. Many group plans will continue to pay for any conditions that are related to the cause of disability for up to twelve months. Again, read your handbooks. A word of caution! In most cases you must request the "extension" in writing, and a doctor's statement of disability must be on record *in the claims office.* Further, letting your health insurance claims office know of your disability may *not* qualify you for the life disability extension. Separate forms generally are required. Disability extension's *group life benefits* can be renewed each year by proving continuing disability.

Once you have been granted your "extensions," you will not have to pay premiums to your employer or the insurance company. You will *only* be covered for medical bills *related to the cause of disability.* Once the months allowed in your extension have been used up, you lose the benefits, unless you previously exercised your conversion rights (at the time you terminated employment or after COBRA's eighteen months).

This may be your last chance to conserve or keep your health and life insurance.

II. HEALTH INSURANCE

Benefits

Maximum Benefits. The maximum benefits your policy provides are usually stated as a lifetime maximum benefit per person. Limits of $500,000, $1,000,000, or even "unlimited benefits," are customary. The larger the maximum, the higher the benefits that can be paid out in claims.

Usual, Customary, and Reasonable. Most medical plans pay benefits according to a usual, customary, and reasonable scale. A "usual" fee is the price usually charged by a physician for a given service. A fee is "customary" when it is within a range of charges made by other similar physicians in your area. A fee is "reasonable" when it is within the above ranges and is justifiable based upon the need for the treatment of your condition. If a doctor charges more than this, the balance will not be paid by the insurance company. Of course, some companies' usual and reasonable fee limits are more reasonable than others. Don't be afraid to ask your physician for the technical name of the procedure. You can then call your insurance company claims office and see if the doctor's fee is within their limits. If not, you might negotiate a lower fee with your doctor. If your insurance company cuts back their benefits (pays less than the full 80 or 100 percent you expect), you can appeal your claim to the company.

Deductible. Almost all plans provide for a "deductible," an amount you must pay before the insurance company will pay any benefits. Your deductible may be $100, $250, or even larger. You usually must meet a new deductible each calendar year before benefits can be paid. Often there is a three-month, year-end carryover. If you haven't reached the deductible by October 1, any expenses incurred during October, November, and December can be used to meet the next year's deductible.

Co-insurance. The co-insurance clause tells you what percentage of your bills the insurance company will pay and the percentage of the bills you must pay. Usually the insurance company will pay 80 percent of all claims (after the deductible). You will pay the remaining 20 percent. In many plans the 20 percent you must pay stops when claims reach a certain level. This is known as the "stop-loss" point.

Stop-loss. Comprehensive insurance plans will usually pay 100 percent of the cost for medical care after you have been paid a certain level of benefits. This "stop-loss" provision usually starts after expenses reach $2,500 or $5,000 during the year. Once your claims reach this point, the insurance company will pay 100 percent of all additional bills that would have been paid at the 80 percent level before. The next calendar year you may have to start over again.

Hospital Room and Board/Intensive Care. Some plans pay only a specified room rate per day, even if the hospital charges more. If so, your plan will state a set dollar amount they will pay per day for semi-private room, or three times the average daily rate for intensive care. Other plans will pay the usual and customary hospital room rate for semi-private, and the usual and customary rate for intensive care charges.

When hospitalized with HIV-related infections, individuals are placed in isolation rooms. This is to protect you from exposure to the various infections that abound in hospitals. There are extra charges for this service. Some plans will pay this extra charge without comment; others will not cover it at all, or will require special documentation from the doctors and hospital that there was a "medical need" for such a room. If such expenses are not paid automatically, call the claims department and explain that you required an isolation room because of your medical condition and ask them to review your claim. Your doctor may need to write to your carrier verifying the medical need for isolation. You can always appeal your claim to the proper state agency. (See "Problems and Complaints: Possible Courses of Action.")

Surgery: Scheduled/Non-scheduled. Most plans will pay for any surgery claims falling within their usual, customary, and reasonable limits. However, some plans will only pay a pre-set amount for any surgery regardless of what the doctor charges. If your plan pays at the usual and customary rate and still does not fully cover an item at the proper level, you can then appeal the decision to the company's claims examiner. Often with additional support information from your doctor/surgeon, the company will pay the balance due. If not, see if your doctor will lower his or her charge to the level acceptable to the insurance company.

Psychiatric Coverages. *Read this section of your coverage carefully.* Many persons with AIDS use mental health benefits. Most plans offer good coverage for psychiatric care during hospitalization, but offer only limited coverage for treatment when an individual is not hospitalized.

It is common for a plan to pay only 50 percent of the usual and customary rate for psychological treatment out of the hospital. There may be an additional limitation of $10, $20, or $25 maximum payment per visit and a limit of one visit per week. Check with your local AIDS organizations. They may offer individual and/or group counseling at little or no cost.

Exclusions and Limitations. All policies have exclusions (things not covered) and limitations (things only partially covered) automatically written into them. Read the excluded list of services carefully to become familiar with the items that may not be covered under your plan.

Pre-existing Conditions. An illness or condition which existed and was treated, or which should have been treated before coverage started, is a pre-existing condition.

Home Health-Care Expense Coverage. Today, companies often include this benefit in their plans. It allows payment for care provided by an "authorized home health-care agency" that starts within a specified number of days after a hospital confinement. This at-home care is usually limited to a maximum number of visits or days (100 to 120) per year.

Home health-care services include some or all of the following: part-time nursing care, home health aide services, physical therapy, medical supplies, drugs and medications prescribed by a doctor, and laboratory services. Read this provision carefully. If you and your physician agree to use such a service, contact your claims department to obtain detailed information and authorization.

Hospice Benefits. Hospice is a coordinated plan of home and in-patient care for terminally ill persons (during the last six months of life) and the family unit. Policy benefits are expanded to include such things as: medical care providers, homemakers, and mental health and bereavement counselors. Hospice care must be approved by the insurance company or plan.

Patient Care Management. Insurance carriers frequently offer the services of patient care management. Patient care management is a concept of "total management of individuals with very large claims." Care management is usually coordinated by a Registered Nurse (R.N.). The R.N. reviews your claims, medical files, and medical history to determine the proper level of services that are most beneficial to your needs. When this benefit is available, services can often be provided that normally are outside the scope of your insurance plan. This service may include home care, health aids, nurses, special beds and medical supplies, and hospice benefits. Check with your insurance claims office to determine if you are eligible for this benefit.

Restricted Lists of Medical Care Providers

- PPOs—Panel Provider Organizations
- IPAs—Individual Practice Associations
- HMOs—Health Maintenance Organizations.

These are examples of medical plans that place some limits on your ability to exercise total free choice of health-care providers. In order to receive full benefits (in some cases, any coverage), you must select facilities and professionals from a selected group or list. It is important to understand your policy features and limitations.

Occasionally, you may find that you are not receiving the care you deserve or require. With "free choice plans" you can always find another health-care provider; however, with restrictions placed on where care can be obtained, the answers are not so easy. If you are receiving improper care, especially refusal of care and care bordering on malpractice, then you must take action. Document all the facts, time, dates, names, improper care, etc. Present your complaint in writing to the carrier's review board or professional review committee. You may also send complaints to the Medical Association's professional review board. Ask the insurance provider—PPO, IPA, or HMO—to allow treatment outside of the approved channels and to pay for such care. If denied, proceed with your complaints to the above review boards and seek outside legal and professional help.

Claims

The paperwork necessary in tracking your claims can be a real chore. Included in Appendix Three is a flow chart "layout" to help you track your expenses and insurance payments in an orderly fashion.

It is important to fill out claim forms properly and to *keep a copy* of all claims submitted to your carrier. Save everything received from hospitals, doctors, labs, and insurance companies. Bookkeeping can get complicated when some expenses are billed directly to the insurance company and others to you. Only by careful record-keeping can you keep it straight. In addition, having a copy of your claims will help in dealing with the claims department when you have a specific question or complaint.

Work with the same person in the claims department whenever possible. This helps build a rapport and a bond of understanding between you and the claims representative. Every time you have any contact with a claims person *write down the person's name, the date, and what was said*. Once the claims department knows that you keep accurate records, you will have fewer problems getting them to listen to your concerns.

If you are unable to handle your insurance coverage and related problems, ask a close friend, or family member, who is good with figures to help you with this task. In case you are hospitalized, it would help to have someone to bring your mail to you or go through it for you so that all important matters can be taken care of and so that no coverage is lost by accident.

III. DISABILITY INSURANCE

Understanding your disability benefits can be difficult. First, you will need a basic understanding of the terminology used in disability policies. However, there is less standardization in this market than in most other areas of insurance. You may want to review your coverage(s) very carefully before reading this section. In that way you will be able to choose the areas of this guide that apply to your coverage. Both group and individual coverages will be explained.

Group vs. Individual Disability Coverages

There are major differences between group disability policies and non-group policies. Group policies may offer short-term or long-term benefits, or both. Short-term coverages offer monthly income benefits for two years, five years, or longer.

Group plans may or may not integrate with public plans (such as State Disability, Worker's Compensation, or Social Security). Some group plans will even reduce their benefits if you qualify for benefits under an individual policy. Individual policies usually do not integrate with public or group plans; however, there has been a recent trend in this direction.

Several states (California, Hawaii, New Jersey, New York, and Rhode Island) have mandatory public disability programs (often called State Disability Insurance). In these states, many group plans offer benefits which start only after public disability benefits are fully used (usually twenty-six weeks). You may be eligible for group benefits if your disability continues after your state benefits have been exhausted. Check with your employer.

Group Conversion or Extension of Benefits in Group Policies

Unlike group health policies, group disability policies may not offer conversion privileges. If there is not a conversion clause, you could lose your ability to file for a disability benefit should you lose your job (for whatever reason) and are considered still able and willing to work. If you are disabled when your coverage ends (because of employment termination), your ability to qualify for benefits will not be denied since your claim to the benefits started while you were covered under the plan. This is generally the case even if you have not met the full waiting period under the plan. Read these sections or the sections on termination and "when your coverage ends."

Since there is often a fine line between being disabled and not being disabled, the question of when to file for group disability benefits may be more critical than for individual policies. It may help to file for your benefits as soon as you feel it would be prudent to do so. (Discuss the possibility of filing for disability with your physician.) If your job is in jeopardy, you may consider filing for any short- and long-term disability benefits.

Remember, filing for disability will *affect both your group health and life benefits*. Review the sections on health and life insurance; then weigh the pros and cons before filing a disability claim.

General Disability Terminology

Definition of Disability. The definition of disability in your policy determines if you can qualify for the benefits in your policy. There are three general definitions of disability used in most policies. It is not unusual for a policy to use one definition for two or five years and then switch to a more stringent one. In addition, some policies will not pay monthly benefits if you are employed in any other job even if it is a totally different occupation than the one in which you were employed previously. It is therefore important for you to read and understand your coverage(s).

1. **Own occupation.** A sample clause might read... "you will be considered totally disabled if you are unable to perform the main duties of your regular occupation."

2. **Any gainful occupation.** A sample clause may read something like... "you will be considered disabled if you are unable to engage in any occupation for which you are reasonably suited by education, training, and experience..."

3. **Loss of earnings.** A sample clause might read... "if you suffer a loss of income because of a sickness or injury you will receive a benefit based upon the percentage of income you have lost..." There is usually a minimum income loss required of 20 to 30 percent. Often any income loss of 75 to 80 percent will be considered a total disability with the maximum benefit paid.

Residual Disability/Partial Disability. Residual benefits and partial disability benefits are similar. Residual clauses allow you to collect a portion of your benefits based upon how much the disability has lowered your income. For example, if you are earning only 60 percent of what you were before your disability, then you will collect a 40 percent disability benefit.

If your policy contains a partial disability benefit and you are not working full time, you will generally receive 50 percent of the monthly benefit for up to six months. Often, before you are able to qualify for benefits under a partial disability, you must first be totally disabled.

Elimination or Qualification Period. To qualify for the income benefits in a disability policy, you must meet a "waiting" or "elimination" period. A waiting or elimination period is the period of time you must be disabled before you are eligible for benefits. If your policy has a thirty-day waiting period you must be disabled for thirty days before you become eligible for any benefits. You will not receive any income for the waiting period. It is much like a deductible under auto insurance. Waiting or elimination periods generally are either thirty, sixty, or ninety days, but may extend up to one year.

Once you have met the waiting period for benefits, you become eligible for monthly benefits as described in your policy. However, there may be a fairly long wait for your first check to arrive. The insurance company must receive your claim documentation, review the information, and verify it with your physicians. It helps to file early (before the waiting period ends). This gives the company time to review your claim and approve your benefits so your checks will start on time. Remember, your benefits are paid at the end of each income period (just like while you were employed).

Monthly Benefits/Income. In an individual disability policy, your monthly benefit or income will be given as a maximum amount you can collect if totally disabled. You may receive a smaller amount if you qualify only for a residual/partial benefit.

There are many methods of determining the monthly benefit under group plans. If you are unsure what amount of income you qualify for, call your employer or your insurance company's claims office. This information is not a secret. Do not be shy in asking any questions you might have.

Benefits Period. The benefits period stated in your policy will answer the question, How long can I expect my checks to continue? Your monthly benefits will continue until you are able to go back to work (when you no longer meet the definition of disability) or you have received benefits for the maximum benefit period your plan allows. The benefits period generally found in policies varies from several months to several years, or may even continue to age sixty-five or longer. As discussed above, your plan may change the way in which your disability is defined. This could affect your ability to collect benefits changing how your disability is classified.

Waiver of Premium. Most individual disability policies include a premium disability waiver. This clause is triggered generally after 90 or 180 days of disability. Once this occurs you will not have to pay any more premiums on the policy for as long as you are disabled. Some policies will even refund any premiums you paid during the first 90 or 180 days of your disability.

Pre-existing Conditions. Read this section of your policy carefully. The wording varies a great deal among different plans. In most individual policies, any medical history listed on your application, and accepted by the insurance company, will not be used to deny benefits due to a pre-existing condition. In other cases, there may be a two-year pre-existing condition clause.

Exclusions. Most policies have only a few standard exclusions; such as, war, pregnancy, self-inflicted injury, pre-existing conditions, and attempted suicide. Your policy may also have been issued with a *special exclusion rider*, excluding a medical or physical condition that existed before you applied for the policy. The exclusion can only be applied to the specific condition listed in the policy. If you think the insurance company has unfairly denied you benefits under any part of your coverage, appeal the decision to your company and/or to your state department of insurance.

Recurrent Disability. If you are again disabled by the same or related causes within six months, most policies will consider your disability as one continuous disability. If this happens, the elimination or waiting periods are generally waived (you will not have to wait again for the benefits to resume).

Grace Period. All individual plans have a thirty-five day grace period, after the premium due date, in which you can still pay your premiums. Many companies allow a few extra days to pay your premium beyond this date. Remember, *your disability coverage may be one of your most important assets.*

If you are disabled and the insurance company has not yet waived the premiums, make all efforts to pay the premiums when due. If necessary, borrow the money from family, friends, or one of the AIDS organizations. Usually this money will be returned to you under the disability premium waiver clause so you can repay any loans.

Premiums. The insurance company cannot increase your premiums on an individual policy when they find out you have AIDS (or any other illness). Most contracts either do not allow for an increase in premiums, or they can only increase premiums for all persons covered in your state at the same time.

Claims. To file for a disability claim on an individual policy, you must write or call your agent, or the insurance company's service office. Ask them to send you the proper forms for filing a disability claim. Read the forms very carefully. Any information that is incorrect or omitted can delay the processing of your claim. Be sure to photocopy all your forms before they are mailed back to the company. It is also a good idea to ask your doctors to do the same. Paperwork has a way of getting "lost in the mail."

The insurance company will review your claim and decide if additional information is needed before approving or denying your claim. The company may want to call or write to your physician(s) for more information. You may even receive a call or visit asking for more information.

Some companies are good at keeping you informed; others are not. You should not let more than two weeks elapse before following up with the insurance company to find out what is happening with your claim. When forms have gone to your physician(s) follow up with your doctor's office to make sure they complete and mail any necessary papers to the insurance company as soon as possible.

Once you have received your first check, determine for how long your claim has been approved. If the doctor tells the insurance company that you will be able to return to work in three or four months, the insurance company may assume you will then return to work and would then stop your disability payments. New forms would have to be filed, causing trouble that might otherwise have been avoided. If the insurance company believes you may return to work in several months, remember to remind your doctor to inform them if you are going to be on disability longer than first expected.

Filing for group disability benefits can be done in the same manner. However, instead of contacting your agent or the insurance company, you will first be contacting your employer. They should supply the necessary forms. If the benefits from your group policy start after your state disability benefits end, start your application one to two months prior to this time. By starting early you can avoid a possible lapse in benefits.

Since HIV infection is a rather new syndrome, there may be a few problems in getting the insurance company to accept it as a valid cause of disability.

In fact, your doctor may not even list AIDS/ARC as the diagnosis. Most companies, however, will only approve benefits based upon AIDS/ARC as the diagnosis. It may be better if your doctor lists all of your current related medical problems on your claim forms *including* HIV infection as the underlying condition. You do not want to refile for benefits because your pneumonia cleared up and you were taken off of disability, when there is still the underlying problem of a depressed immune system.

Hospital Indemnity Policies

Hospital indemnity policies (they may be group or non-group) will pay a set amount of income for each day you are hospitalized. The amount will usually be between $20 and $100 dollars a day. The benefit will be spelled out in the policy. Generally the checks will be sent either to you or to the hospital. If you already have one of these plans, then look it over carefully to see what benefits it may provide, when hospital benefits would start, and what exclusions might apply. Some of the same clauses that appear in disability policies can be found in this type of policy.

Many people with HIV-related problems will be tempted to purchase a hospital indemnity type of policy since advertising stresses that you cannot be turned down for the policy. Before you consider applying for one of these *review the fine print.* Understand fully how the plan defines pre-existing conditions. Most of these plans come with two-year exclusions for pre-existing conditions. You may not want to waste your money on such a plan.

IV. LIFE INSURANCE

Generally, individuals should review their life insurance policies every few years, or when any major changes in health, financial status, or relationships occur.

Basically, life insurance is a contract between the insurance company and the insured/owner to pay a death benefit to the named beneficiary upon proof of death. Coverage may be provided by an individual or group policy or both. The general terminology discussed below applies to both types of coverage.

Kinds of Life Insurance

Generally, life insurance can be grouped into three basic categories:

1) Whole life/endowment policies—generally provide level death benefits and have yearly increasing cash values and premiums that remain the same.

2) Term insurance—provides protection for a specific length of time (one, five, ten years, or to age sixty-five). It may be renewable, at the end of each term, with higher premiums charged on each renewal. The death benefit may be level or decreasing (mortgage insurance is usually a decreasing term policy). Term insurance is the type generally provided through your group insurance policy.

3) Universal life/interest effective life—a generic name for a flexible life product consisting of an accumulation account, term insurance, and expense charges. The balance of the premium, after term insurance and expenses are taken out, earns interest at a declared rate of return. These indexed interest products offer variable premiums, cash values, and flexible death benefits.

Understanding Your Life Insurance

To understand your group life coverage, it will help to have your policy in front of you. If you cannot find your policy, you should request a duplicate policy from your company.

Owner. Generally, the insured is the owner of the policy. However, the owner can be anyone. The owner of the policy is the person(s) who has all legal rights to the policy and controls it. An owner can determine how the premiums are paid, who the beneficiary is, and can exercise all options within the policy. The ownership of a policy may be changed by asking the insurance company to transfer ownership to another person. (This does not change who is insured under the policy.)

There may be valid reasons to change policy owners. For example, if you need to apply for state or federal support (Medi-Cal, welfare) a whole life/universal life policy that has a cash build-up may disqualify you for such aid. If it does, you may consider transferring the ownership of the policy (by gift) to a spouse, family member, lover, or other special person. *Before changing ownership*, obtain advice from either your insurance company, agent, or lawyer, because the transfer may affect the taxation of death benefits.

Remember, once a policy owner is changed, the *new owner has all legal rights* to the policy, including naming the beneficiary and the ability to surrender or cancel it.

Beneficiary. The beneficiary of the policy is the person or entity named in the policy. The owner may change the beneficiary at any time by notifying the insurance company, in writing, on the proper beneficiary change form. The company must record the change in their files for it to be effective. You may name anyone beneficiary that you wish. A non-profit organization may also be named. If you name an organization, be sure to use the legal name and include the address of the organization on your beneficiary forms.

Remember that the insurance contract is just that, a contract. *You cannot change your beneficiary through your will.* A clause in your will saying that you want your benefits to go to your mother will not be followed if your policy says that your benefits are to be payable to your sister (your sister would get the proceeds of your policy instead of your mother).

Disability Premium Waiver. If this provision is included in your policy and you meet the definition of disability, you may file to have future premiums waived (stopped) for as long as your disability lasts. Exercising this clause requires you to notify the company and file for the benefit. The only change that occurs in your policy is the elimination of premiums. It generally will not affect the death benefit cash values but may affect future dividends.

Cash Values/Dividends. An individual policy with cash values offers a great deal of flexibility. Cash values (and dividends) can be borrowed from the policy to pay premiums, pay bills, or for any other reasons. Several things will occur if you borrow from the policy. The loan will incur a simple annual rate of interest (as stated in your policy loan clause). The loan and any accrued interest charges will be subtracted from any later death benefit while the loan is outstanding. You do not have to pay back the loan at any time. Interest will be added to the loan amount each year increasing the loan balance.

If you cannot pay the premiums and are not eligible for the disability premium waiver benefit, then borrowing against the policy to pay the premiums may be an alternative to losing the coverage. Call or write the insurance company to determine what cash values you may have. Be sure to include your name and policy number with any request for information on your policy.

Term insurance does not develop cash values, but it may pay dividends. These dividends can be used to reduce your premiums. Again, see if a disability premium waiver exists in the policy. Group life coverages seldom have cash values or dividends, but there are some exceptions.

Grace Period/Lapse. All individual policies have a thirty-one-day grace period after the premium is due, during which time you can pay your premium. As long as the premium is received during this period, your policy will remain in force. If a premium is not paid during this time, it will go into a state of lapse (the policy will be cancelled). Most companies will allow a few additional days to receive the premium without question. If you are just a few days past the grace period with your premium, call the company to find out if the premium can still be paid.

If the policy is a whole-life type policy (i.e., it has cash values) and lapses, there are still two options available to you. One is extended-term coverage, the other is reduced paid-up life coverage. Extended-term insurance provides coverage for a period of time that is determined by your age and the amount of cash values in the policy. Your policy has a chart which tells you how long the coverage will be extended. This time period will usually be stated in months and days of coverage (several years of coverage may be provided). After the time period has expired, the policy terminates.

Reduced paid-up coverage occurs when the amount of coverage is reduced and the policy is then made fully paid-up (less coverage with no further premiums needed). Reduced paid-up life coverage is determined by the amount of cash value in the policy and your age. You can determine the amount of reduced paid-up coverage by looking for the proper table in the policy. Both of these options will be affected by any policy loans you have against the policy.

Remember, with your current health problems, you will not be able to apply for a new policy. Ask a beneficiary, friend, or family member to help pay the premiums. You may want to change how premiums are paid. Smaller, more frequent premiums may be helpful. If none of the above options is helpful, ask the insurance company to lower the amount of coverage. You will be reducing your premiums and reducing your coverage. However, some coverage is better than none at all.

Cash surrender. An individual life policy with cash values, dividends, or both, can be surrendered for the cash built up in the contract. Ask your insurance company to determine what the surrender value will be. Any of the options discussed above would be preferable to reducing or dropping coverage you might not be able to replace later.

Cancellation. Except for non-payment of premiums, individual life policies cannot be cancelled by the insurance company. The current nature of your health is not cause for the insurance company to cancel the policy.

Conversion of Decreasing Term Insurance. Decreasing term insurance policies generally allow you to change your policy from a decreasing death benefit policy to a whole life policy with level (non-decreasing) benefits. It is often advisable to convert your policy when there is a change in your health that would prevent you from obtaining more coverage. If you convert your policy, the premiums will increase but your coverage will not decline. Check with your company to see how your conversion rights might benefit you.

Amount of Coverage. Group life death benefits will usually be stated in dollar amounts. However, benefits may be set in relation to your salary (i.e., twice your annual salary), or based upon occupational classes.

Beneficiary. When you started to work with your current employer, you filled out your group insurance papers. At that time you listed a beneficiary for your group life coverage. Check with your employer to see that this is still listed the way you wish. Filling out a beneficiary change form is one way to make sure that your beneficiary is correct. Remember, you can name any person, persons, or organizations you wish as beneficiary.

Disability or Termination of Coverage. Either a disability or a termination of employment can affect your coverage. If either of these occur, check with your employer about your group insurance. You may be eligible for a disability premium waiver (if one is included in your group policy). If not, you will be eligible for a group life conversion policy. There may be ways to keep the coverage in force by working with your employer (paying your employer for the premiums yourself). Remember, if you exercise a disability extension, you will generally not need to convert your group life policy.

Conversions. All group life policies have a conversion clause in the contract. If coverage terminates because you are disabled (and your group coverage does not have a disability premium waiver or extension feature) and there is termination of employment, or layoff, you must be offered a conversion policy. You can apply for any whole life policy the group carrier offers as long as the amount of coverage is not greater than the amount you had under the group policy. You must apply for your conversion policy within thirty-one days of your termination date. You *cannot* be denied a conversion because of poor health. However, the policy will not include optional features.

PROBLEMS AND COMPLAINTS

Possible Courses of Action

Poor Service, Claim Delays, Frequent Errors. Call and/or write to claims manager. Document fully and be well prepared and orderly in presenting information. Include names, dates, promises, photo copies, etc. Seek advice from your agent, insurance counselor, employer, personnel office, etc.

Underpayment of Claims, UCR Cuts, Contractual Provision Questions, Denials of Claims. Review, understand, and clarify your coverages and limitations. Review denials and UCR cuts with your health-care providers. Obtain additional documentation from doctors, etc. Write to insurance carrier asking for a formal review, then ask for outside medical review or arbitration. Call for professional help: agent, insurance counselor, legal advisor. File a formal complaint with carrier regulator and/or state Department of Insurance (DOI).

Pre-existing Conditions, Policy Cancellations. Review facts, policy benefits, limitations, all documents. Ask carrier to put reasons for action into a letter. Get records from doctor, agent, insurance carrier, etc. Get outside help: agent, insurance counselor, attorney. File formal complaints with regulatory bodies. Ask for outside Medical Association review.

Denials of Applications (for healthy individuals). In writing, ask the insurance company to release *to your physician* exact reasons why you were declined. Review information with doctors, agent, insurance counselor, attorney. Complain to CIPHR, ACLU, NGRA, Lambda, regulatory bodies.

Continuation of Coverage/Extensions/Conversion Denials. Review policy, documentation, records. Seek immediate outside help: insurance counselor, attorney, agent, or state Department of Insurance.

The above guide lists suggested courses of action. The potential problems indicated should dictate what actions should be taken. It is important to fully understand your policy benefits and its limitations. Many problems arise because the insured assumes "everything" is covered under their policy and the policy will pay 100 percent of all claims. Reality dictates otherwise. With the widespread introduction of plans restricting or limiting health-care providers to a specific list, more people face cutbacks in benefits when the list is not adhered to. Not following utilization and preauthorization reviews will lead to further cutbacks in benefits.

Conclusion

This chapter is not intended to offer legal advice, but rather to help you review and better understand any insurance coverages you may have. Any concerns you may have about your coverage(s) should be discussed with a knowledgeable person.

Section Eight

A Spiritual Perspective

Editors: Rabbi Jeffrey A. Perry-Marx, Rev. Steven D. Preston,
Rev. Tom Reinhart-Marean, and Andy Rose

In the face of the tremendous suffering and anxiety, and the pervasive social
paranoia and stigmatization caused by the AIDS crisis, there is a need for
spiritual and moral leadership. The ignorance which pronounces AIDS as God's
judgment must be answered with the truth of God's compassionate stand with
those who suffer.

"Mobilizing Religious Leaders and Resources"

Living With AIDS: Spiritual Issues and
   Resources

Biblical Perspectives on AIDS

Pastoral Care Issues and Suggestions

What can the Community of Faith Do?

Mobilizing Religious Leaders and Resources

This section was prepared by a writing team of the Spiritual Advisory Committee for APLA:
Rev. Brad Anderson (Metropolitan Community Church); Frank Carusi (Religious Science); Rev.
Wayne Christiansen (Lutheran); Rev. Bill Leeson (Episcopal); Rabbi Jeffrey A. Perry-Marx (Jewish); Rev. Steve Pieters (Metropolitan Community Church); Rev. Steve Preston (Baptist); Rev.
Tom Reinhart-Marean (United Methodist); and Andy Rose (Jewish, APLA staff liaison).

Living with AIDS: Spiritual Issues and Resources

Introduction

No disease of the twentieth century has provoked such violent religious reactions as has AIDS. Unfortunately, most of the religious voices seem to come out of the Middle Ages. Clerics then said the bubonic plague was a result of unholy living, and many today are shouting that AIDS is God's judgment on deserving sinners.

One of the most damaging results of this attitude is alienation. When God is seen as a sadistic torturer who inflicts pain and suffering on us, our natural reaction is to run the other way. The anger of *Why did God do this to me?* is an understandable reaction. But if we don't own the anger and use it creatively, it distances us from God and from our spiritual care-givers. It also creates a sense of powerlessness and victimization that makes it much more difficult to call upon our own spiritual resources, as well as the power of God, to sustain us.

Many contemporary Jewish and Christian teachings do not assert that God is the source of evil (including illness), nor that God uses illness to punish or afflict people. For all of human history, the God of the Jewish and Christian

Contains extracts from *AIDS: Is It God's Punishment?* Adapted for this article with the permission of the Universal Fellowship of Metropolitan Community Churches.

traditions is the One who has sought our freedom from sin, illness, and destruction—not to bring them upon us. This God is the source of goodness. God stands *with* the ill and oppressed, and in true compassion is the One who suffers *with* us in our pain and alienation.

AIDS is not God's judgment on anyone. God suffers with us in this crisis. Those who are clergy, or members of a community of faith have a vital role to play. It is up to you to embody God's love and care for people with AIDS or ARC and their loved ones. When the question is asked, *Where are God's hands in this?* you must answer, *My hands are God's hands.*

Personal Spiritual Issues and Needs

In the Jewish and Christian traditions, persons are created by God as holistic and interrelated beings. Spirituality is an essential part of who we are. Our psychological, physical, and spiritual aspects are closely interwoven, with each influencing the others.

Spirituality has different meanings for each of us, but to all there is the sense that at the core of our being lies our spirit, which while real and present is nonetheless intangible. And that there is a God who, while different and separate from us, is nonetheless involved in our world and our lives. Knowing there is a Power greater than ourselves that can be called upon, can serve us in living a life of wholeness and fulfillment.

When we are spiritually at peace with God, we have a connection with God which brings peace to ourselves, and to our relations with others as well. A result of that state of peace is a real sense of "presentness" with God, with others, and with our self. This spiritual peace is mirrored in the ancient languages of the Jewish and Christian scriptures. In both the Hebrew and Greek, the word for spirit is also the word for breath. Breathing is a taking in and a letting go; likewise, as we take in the presence of God and let go the cares and burdens of life, our spirit achieves a state of peace.

Most of the basic issues of our lives are essentially spiritual issues. Our need to know the purpose of life; the tensions and complexities that arise from our sexuality; the terror and victimization we can feel in illness; and our innate fear and resistance to death—all arise from and are centered in our spirit's relationship to our world and our material being. So, too, is our need to maintain or to reclaim our sense of connectedness to God, to live our life on more than a material level.

When we have left or been expelled from the religious life of our community, we may lose some of that spiritual context within which we desire to live. If we are confronted with an immense problem like AIDS (in our self or in others), we often find ourselves wanting to return to the religious or spiritual community, and searching for ways to come back.

The following suggestions may help you to maintain or strengthen your spirituality, or to reclaim that state of spiritual peace with God, with yourself, and with others.

1. Prayer. We are embraced by God's compassion and love. Seek out that all-embracing relationship by expressing to God whatever you feel (anger, doubt, joy, fear, peace, etc.), and by making known to God whatever you need (reassurance, faith, comfort, courage, healing, etc.). Be specific. Be assured you are heard and loved.

2. Meditation. When active praying seems impossible or inappropriate, and words seem inadequate, it may be helpful to be still, listen, and receive. For example: Light a candle and incense, be quiet, and listen for a message from your inner guidance. You may want to choose a special place in your home to set up a meditation or prayer area. You may also want to set up times of the day for spiritual contact with God, such as morning and evening.

3. Affirmations. These are positive statements of the truth about who you are and what you desire, repeated throughout the day. For example: "I am thankful for the healing power of God."

4. God-reminders. These include anything that reminds you of God's faithfulness and of your relationship with God. For example: pictures, flowers, cross or crucifix, crystals, prayer beads, tefillin, tallis, mezuzah, meditation music, affirmations, or anything else.

5. Spiritual Disciplines. These can help us to feel the strength of God within our own being: such regular practices as daily readings, meditations and prayers; keeping a daily journal of our feelings, thoughts and spiritual experiences; private confessions; keeping daily offices or hours of prayer; and religious or spiritual retreats.

6. Ritual, Worship, and Sacraments. Corporate and communal sacramental and ritual ceremonies help us to feel the strength of the larger community of faith, such as prayer services, observance of religious festivals and holy days, holy eucharist or communion observance, and healing services and rites.

7. Support groups. It may be difficult to reach out, but there are many spiritual and religious support groups available, offering love and support.

8. Service. Helping others is one of the best ways to help yourself. When you focus outward, you get the attention off yourself. You have something to offer others because of your experience with life. There are many opportunities to volunteer with AIDS service organizations, and through other community and religious organizations.

Biblical Perspectives on AIDS

Is AIDS God's Judgment?

Is AIDS a punishment or scourge from God? Some would say yes. Indeed, some members of the "religious right" would probably praise God for this tragic epidemic, which is claiming the lives of thousands of gay men and others. The idea that AIDS is a punishment from God is based on three false assumptions: that homosexual acts are sinful; that God causes suffering; and that God punishes sin with disease.

These false assumptions result from a particular way of looking at society, sexuality, and how God works in the world. These assumptions, and the worldview they reflect, are based on the fear called homophobia, and on a tragic misunderstanding of the meaning of God. It is the responsibility of persons of faith to overcome this fear and misunderstanding, to witness to God's love and grace, and to know God's compassion and faithfulness.

Are Homosexual Acts Sinful?

If you are a person with AIDS or ARC and are also gay, developing a spiritual force in your life to help you with your illness and to promote your own well-being may mean integrating your gayness with your spirituality. Many gay people find a need for God's presence in their lives, but, knowing that some religions are very negative about homosexuality, have asked: "What does the Bible say about gayness? Are homosexual acts sinful?"

For the most part, the Bible is simply silent about gayness. What the Bible is not silent about are the many references to God's desire for the creation to be just, loving, healing, nurturing, forgiving, and whole. In the Bible, God is seen as being for the sick, the oppressed, the lonely, the poor, and the outcast. If you are a gay person with AIDS or ARC, the Bible is not a book which condemns you; it is a book which reveals a God who has compassion for you, who loves you, and who stands with you—its message is hope.

The Bible does contain a few passages that have been traditionally understood to condemn homosexual acts, but there is disagreement among some modern biblical theologians about this interpretation of Scripture. For example, the story of Sodom and Gomorrah (in *Genesis 19*), if it deals with the homosexual act at all, deals with rape and not with loving, consenting gay relationships. Furthermore, many ancient and modern scholars think that the sin of Sodom had nothing to do with "sodomy" (an English term for homosexual acts), but rather with breaking an ancient near-eastern mandate to provide hospitality to strangers. For centuries, the story of Sodom has been accepted by many as a condemnation of homosexuality, but the text itself, as it describes either violent rape or transgression against hospitality laws, certainly does not deal with mutual loving, nurturing same-sex relationships.

Passages in *Leviticus (18:22; 20:13)* do condemn homosexual acts but must be understood in their cultural and historical context. The laws of *Leviticus* deal with health, avoidance of idolatry, and sacrificial practices. In addition to proscribing homosexual acts, they also prohibit shaving the sides of the beard, tattooing oneself, women wearing scarlet, and having intercourse with a woman during menstruation. They served to regulate the daily conduct of ancient Israel. Their purpose was also to separate the Israelites from the pagan nations and their ritual, sexual, dietary, and cultural practices; these were seen as part of their non-monotheistic beliefs and cultures, and were rejected as such. Many modern Christians and Jews interpret the Levitical prohibition against homosexuality as belonging only to the historical context of the rest of the Levitical laws.

In the *New Testament*, there are three principal passages that are often quoted as describing homosexuality as sinful.

Romans 1:27: The men, leaving the natural use of the woman, burned in their lust toward one another, men with men working unseemliness, and receiving within themselves the recompense of their error which was due.[1]

I Corinthians 6:9-10: Neither fornicators, nor idolaters, nor adulterers, nor effeminate, nor abusers of themselves with men, nor thieves, nor covetous, nor drunkards, nor revilers, nor extortioners shall inherit the kingdom of God.[1]

I Timothy 1:9-10: Law is not made for a righteous man, but for the lawless and unruly...for abusers of themselves with men.[1]

These passages deal with vices common in the degenerate pagan cultures of St. Paul's time and, once again, do *not* deal with mutually nurturing same-sex relationships. Indeed, the passage in Romans describes dissolute heterosexuals who leave heterosexuality to experiment in homosexual acts purely for the purpose of "burning lust." The English phrases "abusers of themselves with men" in *I Corinthians* and *I Timothy* translate a single Greek word which modern translators believe may have meant a male prostitute or even a male temple-prostitute. The English word "effeminate" in *I Corinthians* translates a Greek word which simply means "soft" or "pliable," and thus "immoral." Many modern biblical and linguistic scholars strongly question whether these passages even deal with homosexuality at all; or whether they deal instead with sexuality of any kind that is simply "lust for lust's sake." In fact, none of these five biblical references deals at all with loving, nurturing, mutually beneficial same-sex relationships. They all deal with coercive, violent, or selfish sexual gratification.

Does God Cause Suffering?

Why do people suffer? All religions have had to address this question. Our world is full of human suffering caused by hunger, disease, poverty, and many

---

[1]These quotations are from the King James version

forms of oppression and injustice. When these things happen, does this mean they are God's will and, therefore, that God wants us to suffer?

While AIDS is certainly a devastating evil, it is not of God's will. It is not "just deserts" for gay men, sent them as punishment. In his ministry, Jesus never punished people with sickness. He healed them. *AIDS is a tragedy, and God suffers with all who are victimized by it or who lose loved ones because of it.*

Bad things *do* happen to good people. We often suffer through no fault of our own, because the world is often an unfair, unjust place. God's created order exists among chaos that is not of God. God does not cause the tragedy, but God does respond to suffering with healing. God heals sometimes through physical restoration, at other times with strength sufficient to grow in the midst of suffering (*I Corinthians 12:9*).

God's healing is described by a woman whose friend had died of AIDS:

He was an abused child, abandoned by his mother. But in the last months, his mother came to live with him, nursing him around the clock. In their times together old wounds were healed, forgiveness was shared, and faith grew. My friend received a healing gift of family and love he had never known.

Even when the injustice of tragedy invades our lives, God's compassionate love can bring good in the form of healing and growth. We can find God's healing touch in our tears of sadness and our screams of anger. We can find God's healing power in the words of love and comfort shared by others. More than anything, we can find God's healing through that inner peace that comes from God's presence and promises. We can know that in everything God works for good with those who love God (*Romans 8:28*).

Is Sin Punished with Disease?

Is God punishing gays with AIDS? This is the kind of question that has been asked for centuries, substituting many other diseases for "AIDS" and many other communities for "gay." Each time some mysterious malady befalls a nation, or an identified community, there is the rush to see if God did it, and if so, why.

If AIDS is a plague sent by God into the gay community, there are some flaws in the plan. Gay women are not likely to contract the illness, so then God would not seem to be giving the same punishment to lesbians as to gay men. And, what of all the other people who are not gay who are affected?

What about all the people in the country of Zaire, with the highest case rate of AIDS in the world, and it has nothing to do with IV-drug use or sexual orientation? Clearly there is no justification for suggesting that God has found the gay community (men only) in disfavor, and has created AIDS as punishment.

If God creates illness as punishment, what about other modern afflictions? Are all women with toxic shock syndrome victims of God's wrath? Or blacks with sickle cell anemia? Or Jews with Tay-Sachs disease? What kind of justice would it be to visit hereditary illness or birth defects on those yet unborn, those who have not yet lived, to sin?

People had similar questions during the time of Jesus. Then as now, many assumed that suffering is a direct result of sin (and that prosperity is a reward for being right). But Jesus challenged that assumption.

As Jesus walked along, he saw a man who had been blind from birth. His disciples asked him: "Rabbi, was it his sin or that of his parents that caused him to be blind?" "Neither," answered Jesus, "it was no sin, either of this man or of his parents. Rather it was to let God's work show forth in him." *(John 9:1-3)*

Jesus then reached out to heal the blind man. We, too, must reject the idea that AIDS, or any other illness, is punishment for sin. We, like Jesus, must reach out with a healing touch. Rather than God's retribution, suffering becomes an occasion for God's love and compassion to be demonstrated. *When people of faith reach out and touch those with AIDS, they can transform suffering into a living example of God's compassionate love.*

Pastoral Care Issues and Suggestions

What Is Pastoral Care?

Broadly defined, pastoral care is the spiritual caretaking of people, both individually and as members of a community. It is pictured in the ancient relationship of the shepherd to the sheep. The shepherd watches over the entire flock in its wanderings and in its pasturing; is vigilant for dangers along the trail; and seeks out the safe waters and the green pastures. The shepherd also watches over the welfare of the individuals within the flock: keeping them from straggling or straying; tending their injuries and illnesses; quieting their fears and anxieties in the face of danger.

The pastoral care of people is like this. Members of the clergy serve to watch over the community of people. Their role is to take the long view on life's journey, while being aware of dangers, pitfalls, and enemies of the community along the way. They seek to nourish and nurture the minds and hearts and spirits of people, leading them to the waters of life.

Pastoral care includes tending the injured and ailing spirits of people as they confront the great crises of life, helping them to draw upon the power and the peace of God. It is a healing art; the healing of the spirit in communion with God will produce an internal strength and stability which can be crucial to physical healing and health. But, even in the face of physical death, this healing of the human spirit will produce a wholeness of being and a peace of heart that makes death a good transition to new life.

Beyond the picture of the shepherd and the sheep, however, pastoral care also involves the preparation of people for self-reliance, along with reliance on the community and on God. And pastoral care at its best includes the marshalling of the community's people and resources in a positive and loving response to the needs and dangers that people face.

The tools of pastoral care are many. They include individual counseling, family and couple counseling, crisis intervention, home and hospital visitation, teaching and community education, advocacy for those who are unjustly treated, and the example of their moral living and leadership.

What Is the Role of the Clergy?

The clergyperson has an essential role in the pastoral care of persons with AIDS or ARC, their loved ones and their care-givers, just as in any other area of need which calls for pastoral care. Most obviously in need is the person with AIDS or ARC.

Their issues include those of any person confronting a probably terminal illness: denial of illness; fear of death; anger at self, at loved ones, at the community, at God; depression and a feeling of helplessness; acceptance of the illness; desire to conquer the disease. Their needs include: to be in control of their treatment and of their lives; to be accepted by others without fear or condescension; to be understood in their pain, depression, happiness or hopefulness; to be loved by their loved ones; to be touched, embraced, and caressed by people who really care.

In addition, however, the person with AIDS or ARC is usually confronted with the paranoia of the community, and is often stigmatized by the community. This person will often find himself or herself battling negative reactions against homosexuality, and being depersonalized by others as "one of those people who are getting what they deserve." Unfortunately, this attitude most often comes from and is reinforced by members of religious communities.

Another pastoral care issue will often be the relative youth of the person with AIDS or ARC, since the vast majority to date are in their twenties, thirties, and forties—the "prime of life" which our culture values so highly. In our society it is not easy to face death as a young person, or to face the death of a young person.

How then can the religious and spiritual leader best serve both the individual and the community in this crisis of AIDS? What are the responsibilities? Some suggestions to consider are:

1. Educate yourself about AIDS and ARC. Acquire and continually update your knowledge of the medical, psychological, and research facts. Rely on knowledgeable sources of information, such as AIDS service organizations, public health departments, or the Computerized Aids Information Network. Your fears and biases, as well as the community's, can only be answered constructively with the truth about AIDS.

2. Pray and meditate on your own heart's response to the people who have AIDS or ARC, and to the groups of people most at risk. In your own quiet moments, seek out the roots of your own fears of illness, death, sexuality, and "differentness" in others. You will not successfully help others with this illness unless you have truthfully confronted and begun to change your own negative stereotypical reactions. And you will not be able to help people in the community do what you have not done yourself.

3. Make yourself available. Become a spiritual resource person with your local AIDS service organizations, or through the public health department if there are no provider organizations locally. Find out from them what you can do as a religious or spiritual leader. Offer to provide pastoral care for people with AIDS or ARC and their loved ones and care-givers. In your own community of faith, let it be known that you are available to your own people for direct pastoral care of people with AIDS or ARC, and for the care of those with fears and anxiety about AIDS.

4. Begin to talk about AIDS. Make positive use of AIDS-related issues in sermons and in teaching situations within your community of faith; begin to teach loving and compassionate responses to AIDS and to people with AIDS. Find ways to incorporate AIDS-related issues in your religious education program. If materials do not exist, consider creating them; share them with other clergy and with your local AIDS service organizations and public health department.

5. Be willing to confront the issues of suicide. In the context of your own faith-tradition, carefully work through your own religious convictions about the issue of suicide in the face of life-threatening illness. Be willing to work through the issue with people with AIDS or ARC and their loved ones; be present with them in their struggle.

6. Become an advocate within your faith and within the larger community. Seek to educate and involve other clergy within your religious or spiritual setting, and within interfaith settings. Take opportunities to speak out publicly when appropriate, before civic groups and in other settings. Consider being available to your local media as one religious leader in support of people with AIDS. (Also consider coordinating this effort with your local AIDS service organization, so a unified voice can be heard by the local media.)

7. Include AIDS-support activities and AIDS-education programs as part of the ministry/rabbinate and planning of your community of faith. Consider ways to mobilize sensitive and supportive members as part of your pastoral care. Call your professional ministry and rabbinate peers to positive involvement by your own example of loving advocacy. Call the community around you to reassess its response and become involved by your own example of knowledge and persuasion.

What Can the Community of Faith Do?

The community of faith stands in a unique position to assist people in crisis. When that community of faith exists on a basis of sharing God's unconditional love, compassion, and faithfulness among its own members and with the society at large, tremendous spiritual and emotional resources are available. And when that community of faith prizes truth, it is in a position to seek out truth in the midst of ignorance and paranoia, and to share that truth lovingly with others.

The community of faith can exert corporate leadership within society in much the same way that clergymembers can, only with many more and diverse voices. The effect on people in society when their neighbors, co-workers, and social acquaintances show personal knowledge and leadership in the face of an epidemic of illness (and of fear) can be remarkable. It can lead to the lessening of paranoia and the mobilization of the entire society's resources.

The clergy can only do so much, and without support from the people can only go so far. Within the community of faith, it is the support and assistance of the people that is the most essential. In the final analysis, it is up to the people of the community of faith to follow the lead of their clergy, and even to take the lead themselves.

The community of faith should provide an open welcome to persons with AIDS or ARC, and to their loved ones and care-givers. Since some persons with AIDS, or ARC, are physically disabled by their illnesses, physical barriers at places of worship and at meetings should be mitigated; ramps should be installed, doors widened, and some pew-rows shortened to allow wheelchair access without sitting in the aisle.

There is no evidence that AIDS is transmitted through casual contact. Precautions, if any, should be based on reliable medical information, not on ill-informed fears. The virus is very fragile and short-lived outside the human body. Unlike hepatitis A, AIDS is not transmitted through food preparation; there should be no fear of eating food prepared by persons with AIDS, or ARC—in restaurants or at potluck dinners.

There may be legitimate general health concerns regarding the use of the common cup for communion, but AIDS should not be one of those concerns. While other illnesses may be transmitted through the common cup, the alcohol in sacramental or ritual wine kills the AIDS virus on contact.

There is no need to segregate people with AIDS or ARC in worship or other religious settings. People with colds, flu, or other illnesses should exercise the same precautions around a person with AIDS, or ARC, that they would with anyone else. Special precautions or procedures for children or adults in nurseries or religious education classes should be taken only on an individual basis and only with proper medical advice; blanket rules or precautions are not necessary, and only serve to increase paranoia.

Support groups within your community of faith may be appropriate. Consider groups not only for people with AIDS or ARC, but also for those who love them, and those who render care to them. But include these people in the general life of the community of faith as well; don't treat them as modern-day lepers and shunt them off to the side.

The community of faith might also consider providing financial and material support to local AIDS service organizations. Money is especially needed in every community for direct support to persons with AIDS or ARC who have not yet qualified for public assistance or social security but have lost employment. The necessities of life—such as food and clothing—are also needed. Transportation to medical appointments, shopping, or visiting friends and family is often needed.

And there is always a need for friends—buddies—who will be available and will provide emotional and spiritual support to someone with AIDS or ARC and their loved ones.

The Role of the Laity

"None of us is free, until all of us are free."

Whether you have a diagnosis of AIDS/ARC or not, this epidemic affects each of us on an individual, personal level. It forces us to confront our own views and fears about illness, sexuality (including homosexuality), death, spirituality, suicide, and a wide range of issues that many of us deny.

As we challenge ourselves to personal growth in these areas, we take our first steps as individuals responding to the AIDS crises. While each of us has a ministry or rabbinate to do, the nature of your ministry or rabbinate can only be determined by you. The strong, diverse, creative, and inspired response to the AIDS epidemic which we have already seen is the result of various gifted *individuals* who have acted. What does the future hold for you; or rather, what do you hold for the future?

As you contribute to the healing process, it is imperative to educate yourself about AIDS, from responsible publications and organizations, learn about its history, transmission, medical treatment, psychosocial aspects, etc. Periodic updates are also advised. Not only does this education eliminate unnecessary fears that you may be feeling, it can also better prepare you to deal with others who approach you with their fears and concerns. Equally important, acquainting yourself with the facts about AIDS will enable you to better determine the area of your own special and unique involvement.

We each have an individual role in assuring that people with AIDS or ARC are not neglected, abandoned, or judged. In relating to people with AIDS or ARC and their loved ones and friends, take time to listen. Listen to the troubles and the pain; listen to the joys and high points of life. Listen as others share their lessons learned; the turning points; the significant people that have influenced their lives; the transitions, transformations, and wounds still to be healed. Recognize the gifts and strengths possessed by people with AIDS or ARC, their loved ones and friends, as well as your own gifts, as we help each other to heal.

Our prayers, worship, and spirituality serve to bring us into greater awareness of ourselves and all that is around us. We are encouraged simply to be ourselves, as we acknowledge pain, suffering, and loss, yet affirm life. Denial, anger, bargaining, and depression are no longer words on a page, but are real-life battles *we* now are facing, whether as a person with AIDS or ARC, their loved one, or a care-giver, as we move toward resolution and acceptance.

In the midst of all this, it is essential that you care for yourself—your own physical, emotional, and spiritual well-being—for you are truly priceless in your service. Take the time to heal your wounds, to nourish yourself, to relax at sunset, and to share both your laughter and your tears with your friends. Seek out the emotional and spiritual support which you need as you help to provide it for others. We are all in this together, and no one is saying it will be easy. You must take the time you need to laugh, or to cry, in the confidence that there are others involved who are as compassionate and committed as you, and in the confidence that God is there with you.

Some suggestions for individual involvement are:

1) Volunteer time at a local AIDS service organization.

2) Financially support local AIDS research or patient relief and services.

3) Be present with a person with AIDS or ARC; be a companion.

4) Be a patient advocate; legal, financial, and medical bureaucracies can be overwhelming.

5) Help with household tasks, chores, errands, and transportation.

6) Create a pleasant environment for a person with AIDS or ARC.

7) Share a good laugh with a person with AIDS or ARC, or their loved ones.

Mobilizing Religious Leaders and Resources

Organized religion wields tremendous influence and power in society. And it can marshal enormous resources of personnel (paid and volunteer), money, and institutions to meet social needs, often more quickly and more efficiently than government agencies and programs can.

While the various religions are organized in many different ways, almost all function with some form of central leadership. That leadership may be vested in individuals (such as bishops, presbyters, regional directors), in collective bodies (such as councils, conferences, synods), or in combinations of individual and collective leadership bodies.

In some religions, the central leadership figures and bodies exercise direct authority and control over subordinate units. In some, they act only to facilitate or advise locally autonomous congregations; and in others, there is a combination of limited central control and limited local autonomy.

But in most settings, central leadership figures and bodies exercise great influence among the constituent congregations, and often serve to spark or enable the development of efforts to meet unmet needs. In the AIDS crisis, efforts must be undertaken to mobilize religious leaders and the resources of religious institutions to meet the needs of persons with AIDS or ARC, of their loved ones, and of a fearful society.

In addition to the earlier suggestions for clergy, the following are some suggested ways of mobilizing religious leaders and institutional resources:

1. **Educate and advocate your own religious leadership** (locally, regionally, and nationally) with reliable information about AIDS and those it affects. Provide printed material, resource agencies, and contact persons for them.

2. **Organize interfaith committees** of concerned, informed, and activist clergy and laypersons who can provide a base of support for educational and lobbying efforts within denominational and interreligious institutions. Coordinate these efforts with local AIDS service providers, or organize under the sponsorship of an existing AIDS agency.

3. **Hold conferences for clergy and religious leaders** which not only educate but also provide the means and incentive for mobilizing and networking to meet the many needs that arise from the AIDS crisis.

4. **Sponsor leadership forums for religious leaders,** such as information breakfasts or luncheons, educational seminars, and round-table discussions, with a goal of mobilizing them to further action.

5. **Seek the creation of AIDS liaison offices** on the staffs of religious leaders/bodies and in interreligious bodies, so there is an accessible contact person for information, advocacy, and mobilization of resources.

6. **Approach interreligious bodies** to discuss and implement ways of marshalling religious leaders and resources to combat the social stigmatization about AIDS and to provide pro-active support.

7. **Develop effective interreligious support** systems for pastoral care, by organizing and training pastoral and lay workers to function in an interdisciplinary approach with existing AIDS service agencies. (If no local AIDS agency exists, make its development part of such a ministry or rabbinate.)

8. **Organize religious and interreligious leaders** into an effective and permanent body, which can continue to be a forum for public advocacy and a setting for evaluating unmet needs, and mobilize religious and interreligious institutions and resources to meet them.

Conclusion

In the face of the tremendous human suffering and anxiety, and the pervasive social paranoia and stigmatization brought about by the AIDS crisis, there is a need for spiritual and moral leadership. The ignorance which pronounces AIDS as God's judgment must be answered with the truth of God's compassionate stand with those who suffer.

The cries of right-wing religious zealots to shun and quarantine those affected by AIDS must be answered by persons and communities of faith whose love, concern, and care is shown by supporting and sheltering those whom society fears.

And the love and grace, compassion and faithfulness of God must be spoken loudly and given liberally by the religous leaders of the community in the nation, calling all people by their words and their deeds to impart God's love and compassion to all who are affected by AIDS. Which is all of us.

Section Nine

A Healing Perspective

When we stop focusing only on the external outcome of healing, and pause more often to recognize and surpass our fears and our judgments that limit and belittle us, we will see healing as possible in each moment in our lives, thereby knowing to a greater degree our inner magnificence and brilliance.
"Experiencing the Power of Healing"

Experiencing the Power of Healing

A Healing Meditation

Epilogue: When Someone You Love Has AIDS

Experiencing the Power of Healing

*Jim Geary**

The following keynote speech was delivered at the AIDS Atlanta Fourth Annual Banquet in 1986.

This evening I would like to share with you a few words about healing, grieving, and overcoming barriers. In 1982, a friend and colleague of mine who was diagnosed with AIDS talked to me about healing. Paul was a father, psychologist, and founding director of one of San Francisco's leading counseling centers for the gay community. Paul had tried many traditional as well as alternative forms of treatment, from interferon and chemotherapy, to a macrobiotic diet and visualization work.

I encountered Paul just before he was to leave for the Philippines to work with what he called a psychic surgeon. At this time Paul was literally covered in lesions, and it seemed to many of us who knew Paul that he might not return alive.

*Jim Geary is Executive Director of Shanti Project, San Francisco. This keynote address is reprinted from the newsletter of AIDS Atlanta.

I told him that, in my opinion, he had more faith in his ability to manifest recovery than all of us helpers at the Shanti Project put together. Paul
smiled and shared with me how he had accepted that he didn't know what
the actual outcome would be regarding his ongoing effort to bring about physical healing. He also said he realized that he might die of AIDS, but he
approached his life with an attitude that "anything is possible." He was living each precious moment to its maximum.

Paul taught me how to look at healing differently: to understand that healing isn't necessarily an end result, but a moment-to-moment way of living that
empowers one to be and understand more who one is. Healing can be both
accepting and/or challenging—what we call fate. Healing is a way of living
in which we give definition to ourselves rather than define ourselves through
the eyes of others. Healing can occur through both metaphysical and/or practical thinking.

In my weekly support group for people with AIDS and severe AIDS-
related complex (ARC), members sometimes get seemingly polarized around
the issues of healing and its relationship to attitude. For example, a person
using a metaphysical approach, that is, mind over matter, in working with
his illness, may determine that a person who talks about dying, or who is feeling depressed about his condition, is in fact giving power to that condition,
thus enhancing the possibility of death as a likely outcome. Conversely, a person who is dealing directly with issues surrounding dying and depression may
determine that the metaphysical thinker is denying his or her true feelings and
afraid to look at the possibility of dying from AIDS.

Each of these points of view has merit and something to offer the other.
The metaphysical thinker is correct in pointing out that what we focus on does,
to a large degree, become our reality; yet it is also a metaphysical principle
that what one resists, persists. Dealing with one's fears of dying and feelings
of depression can be disempowering or empowering. Often it is only by becoming deeper in touch with our feelings of disempowerment and helplessness that
we tap into a larger source of personal power.

Healing is, regardless of the success of the outcome as viewed by others,
the inner knowledge of our own ability to deal with what we are experiencing. It is our ability to open to each changing moment and see ourselves anew.

My friend Paul died healing. Healing himself and others of our narrow-
ness of vision. Healing us of our apathetic compliance with what we temporarily perceive as inevitable. How seemingly difficult it is for us to open to that

eternal process of becoming more—for us to begin to see miracles not as other-worldly, but as self-worthy and attainable.

Dave is also a friend of mine with AIDS. Dave told me recently of an image he had in which he saw an enormous door. As he approached and opened the door, he was flooded with the most intense light he had ever seen. As he passed through the door into the light, feelings of health, joy, and inner brilliance filled him. In this real, and not commonly accepted as imagined, moment of Dave's life, Dave was shown a way for him and for us. How seldom do we similarly allow ourselves to enter that light and shine, to feel joy and celebrate our physical and mental well-being?

As people with AIDS explore healing, they expand the perceived limits of our human condition. As helpers to people with AIDS and ARC, we may need to recognize that the people for whom we do service may be more deeply in touch with their own transformative powers than we are with ours. Hopefully, if this does occur, our reaction will not be one of having failed them but a reaction of awe and gratitude for our increased awareness of our own capabilities.

When we stop focusing only on the external outcome of healing, and pause more often to recognize and surpass our fears and our judgments that limit and belittle us, we will see healing as possible in each moment in our lives, thereby knowing to a greater degree our inner magnificence and brilliance. It is so essential that in the midst of this epidemic, we continue to feel.

So many people fear that getting too involved leads to burnout. It is my experience that it is *not* getting involved that leads to feelings of anxiousness, of being overwhelmed, and of eventual burnout. It is through stuffing our feelings of grief, anger, and helplessness that we will fill ourselves with stress, internalized rage, and weariness—not to mention ulcers. Change in any form is hard; the dying of one's lover, child, friend is hellish. We must remember that feeling powerful emotions is not negative thinking. You may need to scream for what seems like forever, or cry till your heart feels like it is being stabbed with each incoming breath. But scream and cry we must if we are ever to feel whole again.

We must also find ways to help others in their grief, remembering that this is sometimes as simple as taking a moment to validate two lovers' relationship in a world that calls them sick, or in listening to the anguish in a father's heart, stemming from a wish that he had told his daughter or son how much he loved them.

Let us remember that in opening to current grief issues we often tap a well of unresolved issues of grief collected over a lifetime; grief of friends and family members who perhaps died years ago; grief past or present; grief of a nation whose penal system attempts to control murder through murder; grief of a state and supreme court that would punish as a felony God's most natural and treasured gift: our ability to nurture and love one another.

It is so easy to compare our grief circumstances with others' as a way of invalidating our own. It is essential that regardless of the cirumstances leading to our grief we take the time and the loving self-nurturance to heal those wounded parts of ourselves. Each of us must find our own way to accept grieving and dying as a part of living. For it is ultimately only by accepting the changing nature of life that we are able to release the past and find meaning and new courage in the moment.

For me, it is also a question of how I want to live my life. At times, it feels easier to live halfway; to shy away from strangers; to reason that I am already doing enough; to allow my own sense of inadequacy to gain the upper hand. But I know this isn't the way I want to live my life.

My dear friend Pete is dying of pneumocystis pneumonia. Pete and I became very close in our weekly support group for people with AIDS. I had also known Pete as one of our Shanti Practical Support volunteers. Pete was different from many people dealing with life-threatening illness in that he always wanted to talk about how *I* was doing. In many ways, with Pete I had found the best friend I had never made time for. Although only in his early thirties, Pete possessed a grandfather-like wisdom and gentleness in which I found much comfort. Recently my friend had his third bout of pneumonia and was placed on large doses of morphine. The Pete I knew and loved disappeared. He became withdrawn, self-absorbed, lingering.

Despite all my years of counseling the ill, I felt entirely inadequate in how to be there for my friend. I so much wanted him to die, as much for me as for him, so I wouldn't have to feel such pain. As Pete withdrew, I withdrew. Each visit with him was awkward and uncomfortable. Finally I realized that part of the reason I was feeling so badly was that I had let the most important quality of our relationship die before Pete did—the quality of honesty to tell Pete what I was feeling. The next time I was with him I told him how I missed my buddy and that a big part of me was hoping he would die. To my surprise and relief, when I told Pete these things, he said he understood. He said he, too, was tired of lingering, of trying to show interest in the lives of others, and of having to say repeated goodbyes.

In that moment I found myself and my best friend again because as difficult as it was, I risked being real. I want to seize each moment, to keep my heart open, to make eye contact, to risk being authentic even if it is painful. I know that living life this way will bring us closer to ourselves and each other. And, in living life in this manner, we will have to, regardless of who we are—board, staff members, volunteers, family, or friends—look at and continue to work on our old tapes of racism, sexism, and perhaps the worst of all, "selfism." That is the belief that we as individuals are guilty, unworthy, incapable, powerless, less or better than our brothers and sisters.

AIDS is not outside of us. Let us stop scapegoating people with AIDS as having less desirable lifestyles and needing to be more socially and sexually responsible than "we"; the "we" being people who don't know if they have AIDS. Let us work in continuing to preserve our liberties, and free one another as we combat this virus. Let's take the terror out of this epidemic by confronting that terror within us. When we hear people who are afraid and ill-informed about the illness, let's seize that opportunity to educate. Let's remember that providing new information while acknowledging one's fear goes hand in hand.

As we open to being gay, bisexual, heterosexual people working side by side, let us celebrate people with AIDS as living, loving, sexual, spiritual, and kindred spirits apart from a life-threatening disease. You and I, dear friends, are the future, and the future is merely this moment of limitless possibilities extended.

A few years ago I spoke with one of our board members, Gary, who died of AIDS. I asked Gary several months before he died what he had learned throughout his illness.

Gary responded, "Love really is the answer." Gary wasn't sure what the question was, but he was sure that as simple as it sounded, love was the solution. Gary staked his life on that solution.

I thank and applaud you tonight for joining me in staking our lives on it. Thank you. I love you.

A Healing Meditation

Bobby Reynolds led the following meditation for the 500 participants at the Fourth National AIDS Forum, a part of the National Lesbian and Gay Healthy Conference, held March 13-17, 1986, in Washington, D.C. Bobby had been active in the development of AIDS service programs in San Francisco, and in the nation, since 1982. He was a board member of Shanti Project, co-chair of the National Association of People with AIDS/ARC, and a frequent speaker on the personal aspects of living with AIDS. Bobby was diagnosed with AIDS in June 1982 and died April 27, 1987.

Please close your eyes, sit comfortably, and begin breathing deeply.

Become aware of the heart beating in your chest. Notice that your heartbeat is calm and regular. I would like you to imagine that the place in your chest where you feel your heart beating is the part of your being that is the most loving. As you take your next breath, imagine that this heartspace is being filled with a warm golden light...a light of love. You can feel your heart pump this healing light to every part of your body. It touches that part of you which feels pain and grief, which feels anger and hurt, which feels fear and sorrow. As this light continues to radiate within you, you are calmed and nurtured and comforted. As it permeates every cell of your body, you are able to realize your own special uniqueness and how truly worthy of love you are. This love within you continues to grow and becomes stronger with every breath. It reaches outside of your body and merges with the love of the sisters and brothers around you.

The power of this love is mighty. In this moment, in this room, our love is the most powerful energy in the universe. And, we can form this energy into a beam of lovelight. With this beam, we can reach out to the fear, hate, and hysteria that surrounds us. We can educate, we can become leaders and role models for the world. We can send this lovelight within ourselves to touch the doubts and anxieties that may torment us. We can use this lovelight to find the strength to face another day, the courage to continue taking risks.

We can help all segments of our society to unite with a common purpose, a very human purpose, to overcome AIDS. We can reach out to those people with AIDS in the small towns and the big cities throughout our country and beyond. We can send them our wishes for healing and well-being. We can give them the strength and courage to stand tall and speak out for their rights.

We can send this powerful beam of lovelight to the hearts and consciousness of the policy makers in all levels of government and business, and we can believe in this moment in our ability to affect change.

And we can affect changes in those we meet in our everyday life. Take a moment now and picture in your mind and heart all those people with AIDS who have touched your life. Look deeply into their eyes, see the part of them that is a playful child, that is vulnerable and needs nurturing. See the God-self, buddha, the wise woman or wise man. See the part of them that is a survivor. If they have died, picture them sitting next to you, holding your hand. Remember the memories you have woven together, the history of your friendship. Take this opportunity to tell them again that you love them, or you may want to say goodbye or to give them another message.

Their image slowly begins to fade and gradually transforms into ribbons of color dancing in the wind; they continue to dance in your heart for all time. Know that we can surround our friends wherever they may be with our love— a healing force that knows no limitations. We can cry together over the pain of our losses. We can scream together our rage over the unfairness. Together, we can share the joy of rainbows, sunsets, the warm glow of a smile. Together, we can share ourselves fully. By not holding back, we become vulnerable. By being vulnerable, we can allow ourselves to heal and be healed, to care and be cared for, to love and be loved. By reaching out to another person to touch another life with compassion and love, we can work miracles.

Take another breath, hold it, and release it slowly.

Know that when you feel low or when those doubts and anxieties arise, you have a place to go, a place deep within yourself that is safe and nurturing and loving. AIDS has disrupted many lives. It has left us with much heart-ache and with many questions unanswered. But know—in every cell of your being—that your loving, your caring, your just *being* there, does make a differ-ence and will continue to be a help to those of us living with AIDS.

Take a deep breath, hold it, and release it slowly.

Slowly, begin to come back to this room. Become aware of the people around you. Feel your feet on the floor. Together, we can face the rough times and we can celebrate the good times. Together we can meet the challenges of this epidemic. Together—for we are a family and we are not alone. Slowly open your eyes and look around you at all these wonderful people.

Bobby Reynolds concluded the meditation with a special request that every-one join him in a song that had been a favorite of his for many years. Recently, it had taken on a new meaning to him and to the people close to him. The song is "Somewhere Over the Rainbow."

Epilogue: When Someone You Love Has Aids

The following excerpt is from the epilogue of *When Someone You Love Has AIDS: A Book of Hope for Family and Friends*, by BettyClare Moffatt.

[Editor's Note: The author's son, Michael Welsch, fought valiantly against the AIDS virus and opportunistic infections (in his case, fungal meningitis and Kaposi's sarcoma) for two and one-half years.]

When a child dies before his parents, no matter what his age, it violates the order of the universe. My son Michael died on July 14, 1986.

He was twenty-eight years old.

He was surrounded by his loving family; by his ex-stepmother Nancy, by me, and at various times during that last month of his life, by his brothers Bill, John, and Robert, by his grandmother from Texas, and by his father. In addition, Steve, his friend and therapist, was there for him, as well as John, his roommate of several years. Friends called daily. Michael was also receiving devoted care from AIDS/Hospice workers, from Shanti counselors, and from Dr. Ainsworth. Yet although he was surrounded with the unconditional love and support he had asked for, still, Michael died.

He died at Nancy's house, a half block from his own apartment, as he had asked us earlier, choosing to die at home rather than to be kept alive in the impersonality of the hospital. He made a conscious choice during that last month, to let his deteriorating body go, and to let himself go to God. It was an agonizing time for all of us. And we will never be the same again.

For Michael did not "go gently into that good night." To the very end, the human side of Michael fought for control, for mastery, for breath, for life—LIFE!—while the spiritual side of Michael, who had made his peace weeks before with death, wanted—begged even—to leave the wasted body on the bed and escape gratefully into "that safe and peaceful place where Gee-Gee and Zacky are waiting for me." (Gee-Gee was Michael's great-grandmother and Zacky was Michael's nephew, who had died two years previously.)

How ironic that in the last weeks of Michael's life, we who had prayed so earnestly for Michael to live—"Michael, dear Michael, child of my heart. Don't die!"—now prayed through our tears for his swift release. Again and again the words rose from my heart, unspoken, "Michael, dear Michael, child of my heart. Let go! I release you to God, dear child."

For he was a child in those last few weeks. At times he was cross, fretful, angry, demanding, imperious. At times he was an eighty-pound baby, frightened, crying out for his two "mothers." At times he was a childlike spirit coming out of a comatose state to thank us all so politely for taking care of him.

Writing these words, I am reminded daily of that difficult time, when all I believed in about life, about death, about love, was put to the test. And if one sentence that I write can help another mother, another father, another brother or sister or grandmother, another lover or friend or health worker to understand the process of healing—yes, healing!—in the midst of the process called dying; then Michael's death will not have been in vain. I believe that just as there are alternatives to healing, like the ones Michael explored so diligently, and which resulted in a much longer life span for him than previously predicted, so there are alternatives available in the dying process itself. What we learned in those last few weeks of Michael's life can point the way for another family going through a similar situation.

For this is still a book of hope. This is, indeed, a book of love. And so I close my eyes and recreate the last weeks of Michael's life, not in despair, but in a spirit of hope; go back to that time when everything within me cried out for help in meeting the greatest crisis any mother can face, the death of her child.

There are montages that flicker before my eyes every time I close them, pictures that stand out with a clarity and intensity that match those last weeks the family went through. John, his brother from Texas, sleeping on the floor night after night, awake in an instant to lead Michael to the bathroom while he was still semi-ambulatory. John and I bathing Michael, and Michael's unselfconscious, childlike trust as he let the strong arms of his brother support him and help him with this most private of tasks.

I remember Bill, strong, reliable, tender-hearted Bill, Michael's oldest brother, faithfully transporting family members back and forth to be with Michael, and running errands for Michael for months. He and his family used to take Michael to Golden Gate Park to lie in the sun. They were there for him for months as loving helpers. And I remember Bill, near the end, consumed by grief for both his son, Zacky, remourning him, and for Michael. At one point he was unable to go up the stairs to Nancy's apartment to tend to Michael, and yet still, still, doing all he could for his brother. And I remember Bill holding me when Michael died.

I remember Nancy reaching out to me, standing shoulder to shoulder with me, holding hands at Michael's bedside when he had been comatose for fifteen hours. And I remember sleeping in a chaise lounge in Michael's room, counting the pauses between his breaths, willing him onward to where it would not hurt him to breathe. We looked down at this body, struggling to hold on to life. "Michael, dear Michael, child of our hearts. Let go!"

I remember Robert, my youngest son, calling daily, telling Michael again and again as we held the phone to his ear, "I love you, Spike." And I remember Michael's grandmother, walking into his room with a smile, dressed in a pastel dress, just off the plane from Texas, with all her love shining through her dear face, and Michael saying to her, "Oh Grandmother, you're finally here. Now I know I am safe."

And I remember Nancy and I, with the help of the Shanti counselor, Karen, resolving old differences and falling into each other's arms saying, "I love you!"

The Shanti counselors and the AIDS/Hospice attendants who came the last few days of Michael's life, cared both for Michael and for Nancy and me. They helped immeasurably, and their devotion and unselfish regard for all of us brings tears to my eyes even now. For every family caring for their loved one at home, instead of in the hospital, I would beg you to contact both Shanti and Hospice. They serve unstintingly with love and practicality.

For there were times we did not think we could get through this last awesome task of caring for Michael at home. There was numbing fatigue, occasional outbursts of anger, grief so deep it could not be, and yet, somehow *was* borne, flashes of sheer terror. Am I strong enough, God, to be here for Michael? Am I strong enough to go through this valley, this shadowed place, with my heart wide open, with my arms wide open? Bathing Michael, lifting Michael, turning Michael, talking with Michael, listening to Michael, soothing Michael, medicating Michael. "Little bird, open your mouth," and his mouth would obey while the precious drops of morphine dropped in one by one, and then he would go off in a space so far from us that we were surprised each time he came back.

"He's apartment hunting," explained Frank, another Shanti counselor. "He goes out of his body and looks around and decides where he wants to be. But evidently," and he laughed, "he keeps coming back to Nancy's house because it's the most beautiful, comfortable place he can imagine."

"Let me sing to him while I'm taking care of him," said Sandy, one of the AIDS/Hospice attendants keeping the night vigil. "That will ease him so he won't be afraid." I looked into the room again and again that night, only to see this beautiful black woman kneeling by Michael's bed, holding his hand, while he slept. Her soft lullaby words went on and on, while the candles guttered into dawn.

Within those nights there was time for me, and I trust, everyone of us, to revise our own feelings about death—time to go through each separate fear and anger and grief about Michael's dying. For although the dying process itself is a hard place inside you that seems to go on and on unbearably, unmercifully, and while watching your child die is the hardest task any of us will ever have to face; still, past the struggle there is death, merciful death, not to be dreaded, but to be welcomed. I said to myself again and again during those weeks, "Death is nothing to fear. Death is a kind friend."

The human spirit is resilient. The human spirit *is* love. Each of us had hourly opportunities to question and to experience the intensity of our feelings and the validity of our beliefs. We were challenged in each moment to *be* the love, the absolute, no-holds-barred, unconditional love that Michael had asked for. We were forced again and again to stretch ourselves to the limit of endurance, to the limit of love as we knew it.

And there were times when Michael himself was luminous. I remember an earlier visit, in June, when he sat by the fire in Nancy's living room, with a shawl around him, and we laughed and talked and were happy together.

For it was a joy to be in his presence and I want always to remember those moments, when Michael was more spirit than flesh, and yet, and yet, more alive, more *here*, more in the immediacy of the moment, than I had ever seen him. We amazed ourselves at those times, at our laughter, at our spontaneous expressions of affection, at our own tenderness and vulnerability and again—peacefulness—as Michael began to let go of his earthly form.

Michael had asked for three things to happen when he discovered he had AIDS.

He asked that everyone in his family be healed. Oh dearest Michael, that has come true! I remember Hedy, the head AIDS/Hospice nurse, leaning over him, whispering to him as she tried to find out what was holding Michael back from release during the last days of his life; what was holding him in this pattern of shuttling between the worlds of life and death, and understanding instinctively that he felt that he had not said goodbye to everyone. "Ah Michael," she said gently, as he looked into her eyes and tried to make his wishes articulate. "All you have to do is say goodbye in your heart. And that person will know that you love and forgive him." An expression of peace passed over Michael's face and he fell asleep.

The second thing that Michael had asked for was to be surrounded by unconditional love. During the last years of his life, everyone he knew cared deeply about him, from his workmates to his friends, to the helpers that attended him, to every member of his family. No one experienced more love than Michael did up to the last moments of his life. And that love continues even now.

The third thing that Michael had asked for was to be able to do the work that was his to do. When I first began writing this story of Michael's journey through AIDS, he was aflame with enthusiasm. He envisioned himself reaching out to others who had AIDS. He saw himself telling his story, unafraid, risking his self through telling the truth about his illness. More importantly, he wanted to share his deepest self in courage and in love. He talked often about the awakening that AIDS had brought into his life, the 180 degree turnaround that had led him into a deepening relationship with God. He wanted to make a difference in the world.

"AIDS is a gift. AIDS has removed the barriers between me and other people. AIDS is the catalyst that has taught me how to love."

He believed at the time that he *would* live. I believed this, too. In fact, there was a time when Michael thought himself to be a failure *because* his physical body was obviously deteriorating, despite all his efforts to heal himself within and without by every means available to him at that time. This trap of spiritual pride, wherein you are "good" if you demonstrate health and "bad, wrong, a failure," if the body does not follow your commands, was a hard lesson for Michael to learn. He went through a time of profound anguish, continually seeking to understand, continually seeking peace at a deeper level, and finally, I trust, letting go of the belief that insisted that healing was limited to the physical body and that not healing meant failure.

"Facts are the enemy of Truth," said Don Quixote. This is a statement that has helped me to understand that Michael's healing *was* accomplished. It is true that the physical body of Michael, after more than two years with the AIDS diagnosis, did, in fact, consume itself. And it is equally true that Michael will live forever—in our hearts, in our minds, in our souls.

I like to think that Michael did, indeed, get his last wish—that of making a difference in the world through telling his story with courage and love.

I remember one of the nights I was sleeping in his room, with the lamp turned down so low that there were only shadows in the room, except for the light that fell upon Michael. Around midnight, dozing in and out of a fretful sleep, the little voice came from the bed. "Mama, Mama," and I roused myself. After I had tended to his physical needs and kissed him and smoothed his hair back from his childlike, cadaverous face, he gestured for the legal pad and pen we used to write down his medications. It was extremely hard for Michael to speak at this point. The Kaposi's sarcoma had taken over the roof of his mouth and his throat so that he could not eat, could barely swallow. He spoke slowly, croakily, urgently.

"Write—this—down,—Mama. Write—this—down."

I obediently took the pad and pen and waited, poised. Michael often dictated his requests to us, and we laughingly said that he would stay in control through his dictation process until his last breath.

I understood immediately that Michael's mind was wandering and that he thought I was still writing the book about his life. He had often questioned me in the last few weeks about some minor points in the book, chiefly those that dealt with the changes that had taken place within him both physically and emotionally, since the book had first been published in an earlier edition.

"Write—this—down,—Mama.—Now.—Write this down."

He dictated slowly, with long pauses between words.

"I, Michael,—am peaceful—now.—Because—I am not—yelling—at my mother—anymore.—Because—I love—and—appreciate—her—so."

I waited, tears streaming down my face, for more. What did Michael have to say that was so urgent that it could bring him back to coherency, however briefly, with such urgency? What words were there to leave the world to remember him by?

But there was only silence.

I touched Michael's face. He was sleeping peacefully. All trace of tension was gone from his face. I did not know it then, but except for a few disconnected phrases, Michael would not speak coherently again.

Yet in that early morning moment, Michael told me what I most needed to hear. That he was peaceful. That his struggle was over. And that he loved me. His message was not for the whole world. And yet I share it with you now. "I love you." As he did us all.

I love you too, Michael. And I always will. Sleep, little one.

You are safe. It's only change. Go forward in love.

Section Ten

Self-Care Resources

Glossary of AIDS-Related Terms

Acquired Immune Deficiency Syndrome (AIDS): An acquired defect in immune system function which reduces the affected person's resistance to certain types of infections and cancers. To qualify as AIDS, the malfunctioning of the immune system must not be linked to genetic disorder, chemotherapy, malnutrition, or deliberately induced medical treatments (as in organ transplant recipients). Although the cause is unknown for certain, it is thought to be a virus (HIV) which is transmitted through intimate sexual contact or exposure to infected blood or blood products. Once immune-depressed, an individual becomes susceptible to a number of opportunistic diseases.

AIDS-Related Complex (ARC): At present, ARC has no "official" definition. Simply stated, ARC is a lesser disease response to the AIDS virus. Some individuals develop a few or many of the symptoms of AIDS, such as swollen lymph glands, night sweats, diarrhea, and fatigue, but do not necessarily go on to develop one of the life-threatening diseases that meet the requirements for an AIDS diagnosis. This makes ARC a very broad catch-all category.

Antibiotic: A substance produced by living organisms such as bacteria, or molds, which can destroy other bacteria. Penicillin is the most familiar example. Some antibiotics have shown effective anti-cancer activity.

Antibody: A substance formed by the body as a reaction to a foreign agent or antigen. The antibody formed works only against that particular antigen.

Antigen: Any foreign substance which causes the formation of antibodies as protective substances in the body.

Antiviral: Literally, "against virus." Any drug that can destroy or weaken a virus. Some experimental antiviruses are being used in research trials to treat people with AIDS.

Asymptomatic "carrier": A person who has an infectious organism within the body but feels or shows no outward symptoms.

Autoimmunity: A response of the body to fight against its own self; a malfunctioning or inappropriate response of the immune system. Some diseases are believed to result from an autoimmune response of the body, such as lupus and rheumatoid arthritis.

Bacterium: A microscopic organism composed of a single cell. Many bacteria can cause disease in man.

Basal Cell Carcinoma: The most common type of skin cancer. It forms in the lowermost layer of the skin, grows slowly, and seldom spreads. It is easily detected and readily cured when treated promptly.

B-Cells: White blood cells of the immune system derived from bone marrow and involved in the production of antibodies: they are also called B lymphocytes.

Benign Tumor: An abnormal swelling or growth that is not malignant and is usually harmless.

Biochemistry: The study of the chemical structure and the chemical function of all living organisms.

Biopsy: The surgical removal of a piece of tissue from a living subject for microscopic examination to make a diagnosis; for example, to determine whether cancer cells are present.

Blood Count: An examination of the blood to count the number of white and red blood cells and platelets.

Body Fluids: Fluids manufactured by the body. Although some of these fluids have been found to contain traces of the AIDS virus, not all are thought to be able to transmit the virus to another person. For example, blood definitely transmits the AIDS virus, but there is no evidence that saliva can transmit it.

Bone Marrow: Soft tissue located in the cavities of the bones. Responsible for producing blood cells.

Butyl Nitrate: See "poppers."

Cancer: A large group of diseases characterized by uncontrolled growth and spread of abnormal cells.

Candidiasis: A yeast-like infection caused by candida albicans which affects mucous membranes, the skin, and internal organs. Oral infections are called "thrush" and exhibit creamy white patches of exudate (inflammatory fluid) causing inflamed and sometimes painful mucosa. Common sites are the nailbeds, umbilicus, around the anus, and inside the throat. Occasionally, it may occur systemically and affect the heart and the lining around the brain and spinal cord. Candida occurs frequently in the vaginal area where it is not associated with AIDS; it is also not unusual in diabetics.

Carcinogen: Any substance that causes cancer.

Carcinoma: A form of skin cancer that arises in the tissues which cover or line such organs of the body as skin, intestines, uterus, lung, breast, etc.

Cell-Mediated Immunity: A defense mechanism involving the coordinated activity of the helper cells and the suppressor cells.

Centers for Disease Control (CDC): A federal health agency that is a branch of the U.S. Department of Health and Human Services. The CDC provides national health and safety guidelines and statistical data on AIDS and other diseases.

Central Nervous System (CNS): The CNS is made up of the brain and spinal cord. The AIDS virus has been found in the fluids surrounding the CNS and is believed to affect the nerves of the central nervous system. Once in the CNS, the virus can cause a variety of symptoms including loss of motor control, headaches, dementia; and vision, hearing, and speech impairment.

Chemotherapy: Treatment of disease by chemical compounds, commonly used for cancer therapy.

Clinical: Pertaining to the study and treatment of disease in human beings by direct observation, as distinguished from laboratory research.

Cofactor: A situation or activity or agent that may increase a person's susceptibility to acquiring a disease, such as AIDS. Examples of possible cofactors for AIDS are other infections, drugs and alcohol use, poor nutrition, genetic factors, and stress.

Colon: The part of the large intestine that extends from the end of the small intestine to the rectum.

Colonoscopy: Technique for direct visual examination of the entire large bowel by means of a lighted, flexible tube.

Combination Therapy: The use of two or more modes of treatment—surgery, irradiation, chemotherapy, immunotherapy—in combination alternately, or together, to achieve optimum results against cancer.

Contagious: Easy transmission of a disease or disease-causing organism from one person to another—directly or indirectly. The AIDS virus is not easily transmitted between or among people; it is only spread during activities that expose individuals to the blood (and fluids containing blood cells, like semen) of another person.

Cryptococcosis: Due to the fungus cryptococcus neoformans; an infectious disease seen in AIDS patients. It is acquired via the respiratory tract with a primary focus in the lungs and characteristically spreads to the meninges (the lining of the brain and spinal cord) but which may also spread to the kidneys and skin. The most common form is meningitis with headaches, blurred vision, confusion, depression, agitation, or inappropriate speech. It may be fatal.

Cryptosporidiosis: An infection caused by a protozoan parasite found in the intestines of animals. Once transmitted to humans (by direct contact with the infected animal), it lodges in the intestines and causes severe diarrhea. It may be transmitted from person to person. While this infection seems to be occurring more frequently in immunodepressed people, one study reports incidence in healthy persons as well.

Cytomegalovirus (CMV): A virus that is related to the herpes family; CMV infections may occur without any symptoms or result in mild flu-like symptoms of aching, fever, mild sore throat, weakness, enlarged lymph nodes. Severe CMV infections can result in hepatitis, mononucleosis, or pneumonia even in non-immunosuppressed people as well as 94 percent of gay men studied, but it is usually mild and self-limiting. CMV is "shed" in body fluids—urine, semen, saliva, feces, and sweat. In the presence of immune deficiency, such as AIDS, it can also affect other internal organs and vision, sometimes leading to blindness.

Diagnosis: Identifying a disease by its signs, symptoms, course, and laboratory findings.

Diffuse, Undifferentiated Non-Hodgkins Lymphoma (DUNHL): A rare B-cell lymphoma that is difficult to distinguish from Burkitt's lymphoma. Its relationship to AIDS is uncertain at present and is being investigated. The DUNHL patients exhibit generalized lymphadenopathy and enlarged spleens. This cancer is usually fatal.

ELISA Test: A blood test which indicates the presence of antibodies to the AIDS virus. (Various ELISA tests are used to detect other infections as well.) The HIV ELISA test does not detect the disease AIDS but only indicates if viral infection has occurred. The test is used to screen blood supplies, is used in certain research projects, and has also been used in specific health-care situations.

Epidemiology: The study of incidence, distribution, environmental causes, and control of a disease in a population.

Epstein-Barr Virus (EBV): A herpes-like virus that causes one of the two kinds of mononucleosis (the other is caused by CMV). It lodges in the nose and throat and is transmitted by kissing. EBV lies dormant in the lymph glands and has been associated with Burkitt's lymphoma, a cancer of the lymph glands. This is the clearest link to date between viruses and cancer.

Etiology: The study of the causes and origins of disease.

Excision: Surgical removal of a diseased part of the body, including cancerous growths.

Exposure: The act or condition of coming in contact with, but not necessarily being infected by, a pathogenic agent.

False Negative: An erroneous test result that indicates no antibodies are present when, in fact, they are.

False Positive: An erroneous test result which indicates that antibodies are present when, in fact, there are none.

Helper/Suppressor T-cells: T-cells are lymphocytes (white blood cells) that are formed in the thymus and are part of the immune system, which has been found to be abnormal in people with AIDS. The normal ratio of helper T-cells to suppressor T-cells is approximately 2:1. This becomes inverted in people with AIDS but may also be temporarily abnormal in people for many other reasons.

Hemophilia: An inherited condition where normal blood clotting is not possible. Hemophiliacs take a blood product called factor VIII to assist in clotting. These concentrates are made of the pooled blood of many individuals. Previously, factor VIII often contained the AIDS virus, but now in the U.S. both factors VIII and IX are heat treated to kill the virus. A few cases of AIDS have been diagnosed in patients lacking factor IX. Because of the high rate of previous infection, hemophiliacs remain a high-risk group for AIDS.

Herpes Simplex Virus I (HSV I): The virus that results in cold sores or fever blisters on the mouth. Like all herpes viruses, the virus may lie dormant for months or years in nerve or lymph tissue and flare up again under stress, trauma, infection, or immunosuppression. There are no present cures for any of the herpes viruses.

Herpes Simplex Virus II (HSV II): A virus that causes painful sores on the anus or genitals. Sexually transmitted, it is the second most common venereal disease. In AIDS, the infection tends to persist and cover large areas.

High-Risk Behavior: A term used to describe certain activities that increase the risk of transmitting the AIDS virus. These include anal or vaginal intercourse without a condom, oral-anal contact, semen or urine in the mouth, manual-anal penetration, sharing intravenous needles, intimate blood contact, and sharing of sex toys contaminated by body fluids. These activities are often referred to as "unsafe."

High-Risk Groups: Those groups in which epidemiological evidence indicates that there is an increased risk of contracting AIDS. High-risk groups include gay and bisexual men, IV-drug users, hemophiliacs, and the sexual partners of any in these groups.

HIV: See Human Immunodeficiency Virus

Hodgkin's Disease: A form of cancer that affects the lymphatic system—the network of glands or nodes and vessels which manufactures and circulates lymph throughout the body to fight infection.

Hormones: Chemicals that help regulate the body mechanisms including growth, metabolism, and reproduction.

HTLV-3/LAV/ARV: The three names previously given for the virus which causes AIDS. Respectively, the three names stand for Human T-cell Lymphotropic Virus-Type Three, Lymphadenopathy Associated Virus, and AIDS-Related Virus. The virus is now called HIV (see below).

Human Immunodeficiency Virus (HIV): The name chosen by a scientific panel of virologists and other researchers for the AIDS virus. The name was chosen as a generic description to help ease the controversy over different researchers giving the AIDS virus different names.

Humoral Immunity: The human defense mechanism that involves the production of antibodies.

Immune System: A system within the body that helps the body resist disease-causing organisms such as germs, viruses, or other infections.

Immunology: Branch of science dealing with the body's resistance mechanism against disease or the invasion of a foreign substance.

Incubation Period: The period of a disease between initial infection and the first symptoms. In AIDS this period can be from a few months to seven years or more, possibly up to ten.

Immunotherapy: Treatment of disease by stimulating the body's own defense mechanism against the disease.

Intravenous Drugs: Drugs injected by needle directly into a vein.

Invasive Cancer: Cancer growing from its original site into surrounding tissue, but not yet metastasized.

Kaposi's Sarcoma (KS): A tumor of the walls of blood vessels. Usually appears as pink to purple painless spots on the skin but may also occur internally. Death occurs from major organ involvement. Originally seen in elderly men of Mediterranean or Ashkenazi Jewish descent and young men from equatorial Africa as a slow-growing, benign lesion, it is now occurring in young men, 80 percent of whom are gay or bisexual, and is frequently fatal in its course.

Latency: A period when the virus is in the body but rests in an inactive—dormant—state.

Lentiviruses: A sub-family of retroviruses that includes the visna viruses of sheep, the equine infectious anemia virus of horses, and the caprine arthritis-encephalitis virus of goats. Most researchers believe that HIV also belongs to this sub-family.

Lesion: Describes any abnormal change in tissue due to disease or injury.

Leukemia: Cancer of the blood-forming tissues (bone marrow, lymph nodes, spleen); characterized by the overproduction of white blood cells.

Lymph: A clear fluid, which circulates throughout the body, containing white blood cells (lymphocytes), antibodies, and nourishing substances.

Lymphadenopathy: Swollen, firm, and possibly tender lymph nodes. The cause may range from a temporary infection, such as the flu, to lymphoma, which is cancer of the lymph nodes.

Lymph Gland: Tissue which is made up of lymphocytes and connective tissue and which produces lymph and lymphocytes. Also called lymph node. These lymph glands, or nodes, normally act as filters of impurities in the body.

Lymphoma: Malignant growths of lymph nodes.

Malignant Tumor: A tumor made up of cancer cells. These tumors continue to grow and invade surrounding tissue; cells may break away and grow elsewhere.

Opportunistic Diseases: Those diseases which are caused by agents that are commonly present in our bodies or environment but which cause disease only when there is a change from normal, healthy conditions—such as when the immune system becomes depressed.

Parasite: A plant or animal that lives, grows, and feeds on or within another living organism.

Pathogen: Any disease-producing microorganism or substance.

Perinatal: Occurring in the period around, during, or just after birth.

Person with AIDS (PWA): A term developed by individuals diagnosed with AIDS to counteract the more negative term "AIDS victim" and the less assertive "AIDS patient."

Platelets: A small, circular or oval disk present in blood that is necessary for the ability of the blood to clot.

Pneumocystis Carinii Pneumonia: A lung infection seen in immunocompromised people. It is caused by a protozoan present almost everywhere but which is normally destroyed by healthy immune systems. By the age of four years, 70 percent of healthy children have evidence of past exposure. The protozoan is airborne, but cannot be transmitted this way to unaffected individuals. Once a person develops PCP, they are susceptible to recurrence of the disease, and the outcome may be fatal.

Poppers: Slang term for the inhalant drug amyl or butyl nitrate that is used as a sexual stimulant. Some research indicates that poppers are immunosuppressive.

Prevalence: The total number of persons in a given population with disease at a given point in time, usually expressed as a percentage.

Procto: Short for proctosigmoidoscopy, an examination of the first ten inches of the rectum and colon with a hollow, lighted tube.

Protocol: Standardized procedures followed by physicians so that results of treatment of different patients can be compared.

Radiation Therapy: Treatment of cancer with radiant energy of extremely short wavelengths, which damages or kills cancer cells. Radioactive elements such as cobalt 60, radium and radon, gallium, and cesium 27 are used to produce gamma rays. Super-voltage machines are used as sources of X-rays.

Remission: Complete or partial disappearance of the signs and symptoms of a disease; or the period during which a disease is under control. Not the same as a cure.

Retrovirus: A class of viruses that contain the genetic material RNA and that have the capability to copy this RNA into DNA inside an infected cell. The AIDS virus, HIV, is a retrovirus.

Safe Sex: Also known as "safer sex" and "healthy sex." A system of classifying specific sexual activities according to their risk of transmitting the virus. Safe-sex guidelines are used by people to avoid high-risk behavior without having to give up sexual activity. Those acts that are defined as "safe" involve no exchange of body fluids—like blood, semen, and urine.

Sarcoma: A form of cancer that arises in the connective tissue and muscles, such as bone and cartilage.

Seroconversion: The point at which antibodies to specific antigens are produced by B-cells and become detectable in the blood.

Seropositive: A condition in which antibodies to a particular disease-producing organism are found in the blood. The presence of antibodies indicates that a person has been exposed to the organism but does not distinguish between an active infection and a past infection.

Spermicide: Any substance used as a contraceptive for its ability to kill sperm. One spermicide, nonoxynol-9, has been shown to kill the AIDS virus in the test tube. It has been used in sexual lubricants and marketed as a method of reducing the risk of AIDS, but its actual effectiveness during sex has not been proven.

Sputum Test: A study of cells from the lungs contained in material coughed up in the sputum.

Syndrome: A set of signs and symptoms that occur together.

T-cell: A white blood cell that matures in the thymus gland. Subsets of T-cells have a variety of specialized functions within the immune system.

T4 Cell: One of the subsets of T-cells that help regulate the body's immune system. These T4 cells, also called T-helper cells, appear to be the primary targets of the virus HIV.

T8 Cell: Another of the subsets of T-cells that help counter foreign agents invading the body; an integral part of the immune system. Also called T-suppressor cells.

Therapy: The treatment of disease; an approach to enhancing and maintaining health.

Thymus: A central lymphoid organ important in the development of immune capability.

Tissue: A collection of similar cells. There are four basic tissues in the body: (1) epithelial, (2) connective, (3) muscle, (4) nerve.

Treatment: There is no known cure for AIDS, but many drugs are being used in experimental trials to determine their possible effectiveness against AIDS.

Treatments for AIDS fall into two categories: antiviral treatments and immune system boosting treatments. Antiviral drugs focus on destroying or inactivating the AIDS virus itself. Immune boosters attempt to rebuild or stimulate the immune system. Many researchers belive that both treatments may be necessary to effectively treat AIDS.

Tumor: A swelling or enlargement; an abnormal mass, either benign or malignant, which performs no useful body function.

Unsafe Sex: see "high-risk sexual behavior."

Vaccine: A substance containing the antigen of an organism which stimulates active immunity and future protection against infection by that organism. New applications of biotechnology may produce different approaches to vaccine development.

Virology: The branch of biology dealing with the study of viruses.

Virus: A tiny living parasite which invades cells and alters their chemistry so that the cells are compelled to produce more virus particles. Viruses cause many diseases, including colds and flu.

Western Blot Test: A blood test used to detect antibodies to the AIDS virus. Compared to the ELISA test, the western blot is more specific and more expensive. It can be used to confirm the results of the ELISA test.

X-ray: Radiant energy of extremely short wavelength, used to diagnose and treat cancer.

Appendix One
AIDS -Related Hotlines & Organizations

NATIONAL AIDS HOTLINES
7 days a week, 24 hours a day

1-800-342-AIDS - English
1-800-344-SIDA - Spanish

NATIONAL ORGANIZATIONS

AIDS Action Council
2033 "M" St. NW, Suite 801
Washington, DC 20036
(202)293-2886
Policy oriented legislative work.

American Foundation for
AIDS Research
1515 Broadway #3601
New York, NY 10036.

Coalition of Hispanic Health & Human
Services Organizations (COSSMHO)
1030 15th St. NW
Washington, DC 20005
(202)371-2100

National AIDS Information
Clearinghouse
P.O. Box 6003
Rockville, MD 20850
1-800-458-5231
*Information on everything from local
organizations to medical research.*

Mothers of AIDS Patients (MAP)
P.O. Box 81082
San Diego, CA 92128
(619)234-3432
or
P.O. Box 1763
Lomita, CA 90717-9998
(213)530-2109

ALABAMA

STATE AIDS HOTLINE 1-800-228-0469

Birmingham AIDS Outreach
2503 Eleventh Ave. South
Birmingham, AL
(205)322-0757

ALASKA

STATE AIDS HOTLINE
1-800-478-AIDS

Alaskan AIDS Assistance Association
417 West Eighth Ave.
Anchorage, AK 99501
(907)276-4880

ARIZONA

STATE AIDS HOTLINE 1-800-334-1540

AIDS INFORMATION LINE
(602)234-2752

Arizona AIDS Project
736 E. Flynn St.
Phoenix, AZ 85014
(602)277-1929
HOTLINE (602)277-1961

Arizona Stop AIDS Project
919 N. First St.
Phoenix, AZ 85014
(602)420-9396

Tucson AIDS Project
151 S. Tucson Blvd., Suite 252
Tucson, AZ 85716
(602)322-6226
HOTLINES (602)326-AIDS,
(602)326-2437

ARKANSAS

ARKANSAS AIDS HOTLINE
1-800-445-7720

Arkansas AIDS Foundation
P.O. Box 5007
Little Rock, AR 72225
(501)663-7833

CALIFORNIA

STATE AIDS HOTLINES:

NO. CALIFORNIA
1-800-367-2437
SO. CALIFORNIA
1-800-922-2437

Northern California:

AIDS Project of the East Bay
565 16th St.
Oakland, CA 94612
(415)834-8181

Ellipse
2121 S. El Camino Real, #505
San Mateo, CA 94403
(415)572-9702

Gay Men's Health Collective
2339 Durant
Berkeley, CA 94704
(415)644-0425

Sacramento AIDS Foundation
1900 K St., Suite 201
Sacramento, CA 95814
(916)448-AIDS

San Francisco AIDS Foundation
25 Van Ness Ave., Suite 660
San Francisco, CA 94102
(415)864-5855

Shanti Project
525 Howard St.
San Francisco, CA 94105

Sonoma County AIDS Network
Face to Face
P.O. Box 1599
Guerneville, CA 95446
(707)887-1581

Southern California:

Aid For AIDS
8235 Santa Monica Blvd., #200
W. Hollywood, CA 90046
(213)656-1107

AIDS Project Los Angeles
6721 Romaine St.
Los Angeles, CA 90036
(213)962-1600

CORE Program
7740 1/2 Santa Monica Blvd.
W. Hollywood, CA
(213)656-8201
Bi-lingual education program geared toward Hispanics and street hustlers.

Gay & Lesbian Community
Service Center
12832 Garden Grove Blvd,
Suite A
Garden Grove, CA 92643
Front Desk (714)534-0862
Crisis Line (714)534-3261
AIDS Response Program (714)534-0961

Long Beach Dept. of Health
AIDS Office
2655 Pine Ave.
Long Beach, CA 90806
(213)427-7421

Project AHEAD
1936A East Fourth
Long Beach, CA 90802
(213)590-9019

San Diego AIDS Project
3777 Fourth Ave.
San Diego, CA 92103
(619)543-0300

COLORADO

STATE AIDS HOTLINE 1-800-252-2437
AIDS HOTLINE (303)333-4336

Colorado AIDS Project
1576 Sherman
Denver, CO 80203
(303)837-0166

Denver Catholic Community Services
Hospice of Peace
200 Josephine St.
Denver, CO 80206
(303)388-4435

CONNECTICUT

STATE AIDS HOTLINE (203)566-1157

AIDS Project of Greater Danbury
P.O. Box 91
Bethel, CT 06801
(203)426-5626
HOTLINE (203)797-7900

AIDS Project New Haven
254 College St., Suite 200
New Haven, CT 06511
(203)624-0947
HOTLINE (203)624-AIDS

Northwest Connecticut AIDS Project
P.O. Box 985
Torrington, CT 06790
(203)482-1596
HOTLINE (203)567-4111

DELAWARE

STATE AIDS HOTLINE 1-800-422-0429

AIDS PROGRAM OFFICE (302)995-8422

DISTRICT OF COLUMBIA

AIDS INFORMATION (202)332-AIDS

Whitman-Walker Clinic
1407 "S" St., NW
Washington, DC 20009
(202)797-3500
HOTLINES (202)332-2437, (202)332-3926

LifeLink
2025 Eye St., NW, Suite 417
Washington, DC 20006
(202)833-3070

FLORIDA

AIDS HOTLINE 1-800-FLA-AIDS

Center One/AID
P.O. Box 8152
Ft. Lauderdale, FL 33310
(305)561-0807
HOTLINE 1-800-325-5371

North Central Florida AIDS Network
1005-I SE Fourth Ave.
Gainesville, FL 32601
(904)372-4370

Health Crisis Network
1351 NW 20th St.
Miami, FL 33242
(305)326-8833
HOTLINE (305)324-5148, (305)634-4636

GEORGIA

STATE AIDS HOTLINE 1-800-551-2728

AID Atlanta
1132 W. Peachtree St. NW, Suite 102
Atlanta, GA 30309
(404)872-0600
HOTLINE (404)876-9944

AIDS Crisis Volunteers
2623 Washington Rd., Suite 101-E
Augusta, GA 30904
(404)733-9000

HAWAII

STATE AIDS HOTLINE 1-808-922-1313

AIDS Foundation of Hawaii
P.O. Box 88980
Honolulu, HI 96830
(808)924-2437

Gay Community Center
1154 Fort St. Mall, Suite 415
Honolulu, HI 96801
(808)536-6000

IDAHO

STATE AIDS HOTLINE 1-800-833-AIDS

STATE AIDS PROGRAM (208)334-5930

ILLINOIS

STATE AIDS HOTLINE 1-800-243-2438

AIDS Foundation of Chicago
2035 N. Lincoln Ave.
Chicago, IL 60614
(312)525-9466

Madison County AIDS
Prevention Program
1254 Niedringhaus Ave.
Granite, IL 62040
(618)452-1380
HOTLINE 1-800-345-2383

INDIANA

STATE OFFICE OF AIDS ACTIVITY
(317)633-0851

Shalico Center
1106 Meridian Plaza
Room 555
Anderson, IN 46016
(317)646-9206

Catholic Social Services
919 Fairfield Ave.
Ft. Wayne, IN 46802
(219)422-7511

Bag Ladies
P.O. Box 441211
Indianapolis, IN 46224
(317)632-0123

IOWA

STATE AIDS HOTLINE 1-800-532-3301

Central Iowa AIDS Project
c/o American Red Cross
(515)243-7681
HOTLINE 1-800-445-AIDS

KANSAS

STATE AIDS HOTLINE 1-800-232-0040

KENTUCKY

STATE AIDS HOTLINE 1-800-654-AIDS

AIDS Crisis Task Force
P.O. Box 11442
Lexington, KY 40575
(606)281-5151

Louisville-Jefferson Co. Board of Health
AIDS Prevention Office
(502)625-5601

LOUISIANA

AIDS HOTLINE NEW ORLEANS
(504)522-2437
OUTSIDE NEW ORLEANS
1-800-922-4379

Central Louisiana AIDS Support Svcs.
1771 Elliott St., Suite B
Alexandria, LA 71301
(318)442-1010

New Orleans AIDS Project
1231 Prytania St.
New Orleans, LA 70130
(504)523-3755

MAINE

STATE AIDS HOTLINES (207)775-1267,
1-800-851-2437

AIDS Project Portland
48 Deering St.
Portland, ME 04104
(207)774-6877

MARYLAND

STATE AIDS HOTLINE 1-800-638-6252

AIDS Interfaith Network
210 W. Madison St.
Baltimore, MD 21201
(301)728-5545

MASSACHUSETTS

STATE AIDS HOTLINE 1-800-235-2331

AIDS Action Committee
131 Clarendon St.
Boston, MA 02116
(617)437-6200

AIDS Project Worcester
51 Jackson St.
Worcester, MA 01609
(508)755-3773

MICHIGAN

STATE AIDS HOTLINE 1-800-872-AIDS

Community Health & Awareness Group
3028 E. Grand Blvd.
Detroit, MI 48202
(313)872-2424

Wellness House of Michigan
P.O. Box 03827
Detroit, MI 48203
(313)342-1230

MINNESOTA

STATE AIDS HOTLINES (612)870-0700,
1-800-248-AIDS

Minnesota AIDS Project
2025 Nicollett Ave. South, #200
Minneapolis, MN 55044
(612)870-7773

MISSISSIPPI

STATE AIDS HOTLINE 1-800-826-2961

Mississippi Gay Alliance
P.O. Box 8342
Jackson, MI 32904
(601)353-7611

MISSOURI

STATE AIDS HOTLINE 1-800-533-2437

St. Louis Effort For AIDS
4050 Lindell Blvd.
Saint Louis, MO 63108
(314)531-2847
HOTLINE (314)531-7400

MONTANA

STATE AIDS HOTLINE 1-800-537-6187

Billings AIDS Support Network
P.O. Box 1748
Billings, MT 59103
(406)245-2029

NEBRASKA

STATE AIDS HOTLINE 1-800-432-7514,
1-800-782-2437

Nebraska AIDS Project
3624 Leavenworth St.
Omaha, NE 68105
(402)342-4233

NEVADA

STATE AIDS HOTLINE 1-800-842-AIDS

AID For AIDS of Nevada
2211 S. Maryland Parkway
Las Vegas, NV 89104
(702)369-6162

NEW HAMPSHIRE

STATE AIDS HOTLINE 1-800-872-8909

Feminist Health Center of Portsmouth
STD Clinic
232 Court St.
Portsmouth, NH 03801
(603)436-7588

NEW JERSEY

STATE AIDS HOTLINE 1-800-624-2377

Hyacinth Foundation
211 Livingston Ave.
New Brunswick, NJ 08901
1-800-433-0254

NEW MEXICO

STATE AIDS HOTLINE 1-800-545-AIDS

AIDS Prevention Program
1190 South St. Francis Dr.
Santa Fe, NM 87503
(505)827-0090

New Mexico AIDS Services
129 W. San Francisco
Santa Fe, NM 87501
(505)984-0911

New Mexico AIDS Services
124 Quincy NE
Albuquerque, NM 87108
(505)266-0911

Southwest AIDS Committee
P.O. Box 6850
Las Cruces, NM 88006
(505)525-AIDS

NEW YORK

STATE AIDS HOTLINE 1-800-462-1884

AIDS Council of NENY
307 Hamilton St.
Albany, NY 12210
(518)434-4686
HOTLINE (518)445-AIDS

Gay Men's Health Crisis
129 West 20th St.
New York, NY 10011
(212)807-6664
HOTLINE (212)807-6655

Western New York AIDS Program
220 Delaware, Suite 512
Buffalo, NY 14202
(716)847-2441
HOTLINE (716)847-2437

AIDS Rochester
20 University Ave.
Rochester, NY 14605
(716)232-3580
HOTLINE (716)232-4430

NORTH CAROLINA

STATE AIDS HOTLINE 1-800-342-2437

Metrolina AIDS Project
1801 Fifth St.
Charlotte, NC 28204
(704)333-2437

NORTH DAKOTA

STATE AIDS HOTLINE 1-800-472-2180

OHIO

STATE AIDS HOTLINE 1-800-332-2437

Columbus AIDS Task Force
1500 West Third, #329
Columbus, OH 43212
(614)488-2437
HOTLINE (614)645-2437

OKLAHOMA

STATE AIDS HOTLINE 1-800-522-9054

OREGON

STATE AIDS HOTLINE 1-800-777-2437

Cascade AIDS Project
408 SW Second, Suite 412
Portland, OR 97204
(503)223-5907

PENNSYLVANIA

STATE AIDS HOTLINE 1-800-692-7254

Philadelphia AIDS Task Force
1216 Walnut
Philadelphia, PA 19107
(215)545-8686
HOTLINE (215)732-AIDS

Pittsburgh AIDS Task Force
141 S. Highland
Pittsburgh, PA 15206
(412)363-6500

RHODE ISLAND

Rhode Island Project AIDS
22 Hayes St.
Providence, RI 02908
(401)277-6545
HOTLINE (401)277-6502

SOUTH CAROLINA

STATE AIDS HOTLINE 1-800-322-AIDS

Palmetto AIDS Life Support Services
P.O. Box 12124
Columbia, SC 29211
(803)779-7257
HOTINE 1-800-868-PALS

SOUTH DAKOTA

STATE AIDS HOTLINE 1-800-592-1861

Public Health Center
1320 S. Minnesota Ave.
Sioux Falls, SD 57105
(605)335-5020

TENNESSEE

STATE AIDS HOTLINE 1-800-525-2437

Aid to End AIDS Committee
689 Melrose
Memphis, TN 38104
(901)458-2437

Nashville CARES
P.O. Box 25107
Nashville, TN 37202
(615)385-1510
HOTLINE (615)385-AIDS

TEXAS

STATE AIDS HOTLINE 1-800-248-1091

AIDS Foundation Houston
3927 Essex Lane,
Suite 1155
Houston, TX 77027
(713)623-6796
HOTLINE (713)524-AIDS

AIDS Services of Austin
P.O. Box 4874
202 West 17th
Austin, TX 78765
(512)-472-2273
HOTLINE (512)472-AIDS

Coastal Bend AIDS Foundation
616 South Tancahua
Corpus Christi, TX 78401
(512)883-5815
HOTLINE(512)883-CARE

West Texas AIDS Foundation
P.O. Box 93120
Lubbock, TX 79493
(806)747-2437

UTAH

AIDS HOTLINE 1-800-537-1046

Utah AIDS Foundation
P.O. Box 3373
Salt Lake City, UT 84110
(801)531-8238
1-800-FON-AIDS

VERMONT

AIDS HOTLINE 1-800-882-AIDS

Vermont CARES
30 Elmwood Ave.
Burlington, VT 05402
(802)863-AIDS

VIRGINIA

AIDS HOTLINE 1-800-533-4148

Tidewater AIDS Crisis Task Force
814 W. 41st St.
Norfolk, VA 23508
(804)423-5859

WASHINGTON

AIDS HOTLINE 1-800-272-AIDS

Northwest AIDS Foundation
1818 E. Madison
Seattle, WA 98122
(206)329-6923
HOTLINE (206)587-4999

WEST VIRGINIA

AIDS HOTLINE 1-800-642-8244

WISCONSIN

AIDS HOTLINE 1-800-334-AIDS

Madison AIDS Support Network
23 N. Pickney
Madison, WI 53703
(608)255-1711

Milwaukee AIDS Project
315 W. Court Street
Milwaukee, WI 53212
(414)273-2437

WYOMING

AIDS HOTLINE 1-800-327-3577

Wyoming AIDS Project
P.O. Box 9353
Casper, WY 82609
(307)237-7833

Appendix Two
Books, Tapes, and Periodicals

The sheer volume of books available on the subject of AIDS prohibits our including all of them. Listed here, by category, are some of the more widely available books. See the Bibliographic References at the end of this section for more information, or contact your local librarian. Most community-based AIDS organizations have free informational pamphlets available as well.

GENERAL

Altman, Dennis. *AIDS in the Mind of America: The Social, Political, and Psychological Impact of a New Epidemic*. New York: Doubleday, 1986.

Alyson, Sasha. *You Can Do Something About AIDS*. Boston: The Stop AIDS Project, 1988.

Antonio, Gene. *The AIDS Cover-up: The Real and Alarming Facts About AIDS*. San Francisco: Ignatius Press, 1986.

Baker, Jane. *AIDS: Everything You Must Know About the Killer Epidemic of the '80s*. Saratoga, Calif.: R & E Publishers, 1986.

Bateson, Catherine, and Richard Goldsby. *Thinking AIDS: The Social Response to the Biological Threat*. Reading, Mass.: Addison-Wesley, 1988.

Benza, Joseph., Jr., and Ralph Zumwalde. *Preventing AIDS: A Practical Guide for Everyone*. Cincinnati: Jalsco, 1987.

Black, David. *The Plague Years: A Chronicle of AIDS, the Epidemic of Our Times*. New York: Simon & Schuster, 1986.

Cahill, Kevin, ed. *AIDS: The Epidemic*. New York: St. Martin's Press, 1983.

Cantwell, Alan, Jr. *AIDS: The Mystery & The Solution*. Los Angeles: Aries Rising Press, 1983.

Clarke, Leon, and Malcolm Potts. *The AIDS Reader: Documentary History of a Modern Epidemic*. Brookline, Mass.: Branden Publishing Co., 1988.

Corless, Inge, and Mary Pittman-Lindeman, eds. *AIDS: Principles, Practices, and Politics*. Washington, D.C.: Hemisphere Publishing Corporation, 1988.

Crimp, Douglas, ed. *AIDS: Cultural Analysis/Cultural Activism.*. Cambridge: MIT Press, 1988.

Dreuilhe, Emmanuel. *Mortal Embrace: Living with AIDS*. New York: Hill & Wang, 1988.

Eidson, Ted, ed. *The AIDS Caregiver's Handbook*. New York: St. Martin's Press, 1988.

Fee, Elizabeth, and Daniel Fox, eds. *AIDS: The Burdens of History*. Berkeley, Calif.: University of California Press, 1988.

Feldman, Douglas, and Thomas Johnson, eds. *The Social Dimensions of AIDS: Method and Theory*. Westport, Conn.: Greenwood Press, 1986.

Fettner, Ann Giudici, and William Check. *The Truth About AIDS: Evolution of an Epidemic*. New York: Holt, Rhinehart & Wilson, 1984.

Fisner, Richard. *AIDS: Your Questions Answered*. London: Gay Men's Press, 1984.

Frumkin, Lyn, and John Leonard. *Questions and Answers On AIDS*. New York: Avon, 1987.

Goldblum, Peter, and Martin Delaney. *Strategies for Survival: A Gay Men's Health Manual for the Age of AIDS*. New York: St. Martin's Press, 1987.

Gong, Victor, and Norman Rudnick, eds. *AIDS: Facts and Issues*. New Brunswick, N.J.: Rutgers University Press, 1986.

Gong, Victor, ed. *Understanding AIDS: A Comprehensive Guide*. New Brunswick, N.J.: Rutgers University Press, 1985.

Gregory, Scott, and Bianca Leonardo. *Conquering AIDS Now!* New York: Warner Books, 1989.

Hoffman, William. *AIDS Is a Play*. New York: Vintage Books, 1985.

Institute of Medicine/National Academy of Sciences. *Mobilizing Against AIDS: The Unfinished Story of a Virus*. Cambridge: Harvard University Press, 1986.

Institute of Medicine/National Academy of Sciences. *Confronting AIDS: Directions for Public Health, Health Care, and Research*. Washington, D.C.: National Academy Press, 1986.

Jennings, Chris. *Understanding and Preventing AIDS: A Book for Everyone*. Cambridge, Mass: Health Alert Press, 1985.

Kubler-Ross, Elisabeth. *AIDS: The Ultimate Challenge*. New York: Macmillan, 1987.

Kurland, Morton. *Coping With AIDS*. New York: Rosen Publishing Group, 1987.

Langone, John. *AIDS: The Facts*. Boston: Little, Brown & Co., 1988.

Leibowitch, Jacques. *A Strange Virus of Unknown Origin*. Translated by Richard Howards. New York: Ballantine Books, 1984.

Llewellyn-Jones, Derek. *Herpes, AIDS and Other STDs*. Boston: Faber & Faber, 1985.

Marteli, Leonard. *When Someone You Know Has AIDS: A Practical Guide*. New York: Crown, 1987.

McCarroll, Tolbert. *Morning Glory Babies: Children with AIDS and the Celebration of Life*. New York: St. Martin's Press, 1988.

McKusick, Leon, ed. *What to Do About AIDS: Physicians and Mental Health Professionals Discuss the Issues*. Berkeley, Calif.: University of California Press, 1986.

Melton, George R. *Beyond AIDS*. Brotherhood Press. Order from IBS Press, 744 Pier Avenue, Santa Monica, CA 90405. (213)450-6485.

Miller, David. *Living With AIDS and HIV*. Dobbs Ferry, N.Y.: Sheridan House, 1987.

Patton, Cindy. *Sex and Germs: The Politics of AIDS*. Boston: South End Press, 1985.

Pierce, Christine, and Donald VanDeVeer. *AIDS: Ethics and Public Policy*. Belmont, Calif.: Wadsworth, 1988.

Puckett, Sam, and Alan Emery. *Managing AIDS in the Workplace*. Reading, Mass.: Addison-Wesley, 1988.

Reed, Paul. *Serenity: Challenging the Fear of AIDS—From Despair To Hope*. Berkeley, Calif.: Celestial Arts, 1987.

Shilts, Randy. *And the Band Played On: Politics, People, and the AIDS Epidemic*. New York: St. Martin's Press, 1987.

Siegal, Frederick P., and Marta Siegal. *AIDS: The Medical Mystery*. New York: Grove Press, 1983.

Slaff, James I., and John K. Brubaker. *The AIDS Epidemic: How You Can Protect Yourself and Your Family—Why You Must*. New York: Warner Books, 1985.

Smith, William Hovey, ed. *Plain Words About AIDS*. Sandersville, Ga.: Whitehall Press-Budget Publications, 1985.

Strecker, Robert. *AIDS And the Doctors Of Death*. Los Angeles: Aries Rising Press, 1988.

Watney, Simon. *Policing Desire: Pornography AIDS and the Media*. Minneapolis, Minn.: University of Minnesota Press, 1987.

PREVENTION/SAFE SEX

Breitman, Patti, Paul Reed, and Kim Knutson. *How to Persuade Your Lover to Use a Condom...and Why You Should*. Rocklin, Calif.: Prima Publishing, 1987.

Douglas, Paul Harding, and Laura Pinsky. *The Essential AIDS Fact Book: What You Need to Know to Protect Yourself, Your Family, All Your Loved Ones*. New York: Pocket Books, 1987.

Everett, Jane and Walter Glanz. *The Condom Book: The Essential Guide for Men and Women*. New York: NAL/Signet, 1987.

Institute for the Advanced Study of Human Sexuality. *Safe Sex in the Age of AIDS: For Men and Women*. Secaucus, N.J.: Citadel Press, 1986.

Institute for the Advanced Study of Human Sexuality. *The Complete Guide to Safe Sex*. Exodus Trust, 1987. Order from Multi-Focus, 1525 Franklin St., San Francisco, CA 94109. (415)673-5103.

Jacobs, George, and Joseph Kerrins. *The AIDS File*. Woods Hole, Mass.: Cromlech Books, 1987.

Kilby, Donald. *A Manual of Safe Sex: Intimacy Without Fear*. Los Angeles: Publishers Marketing Services, 1987.

Mandel, Bea, and Byron Mandel. *Stay Safe*. Rocklin, Calif.: Prima Publishing, 1987.

Peters, Brooks. *Terrific Sex in Fearful Times*. New York: St. Martin's Press, 1988.

Preston, John, and Glenn Swann. *Safe Sex: The Ultimate Erotic Guide*. New York: NAL/Plume, 1987.

Scotti, Angelo, and Thomas Moore. *Safe Sex*. New York: PaperJacks, 1987.

Ulene, Art. *Safe Sex in a Dangerous World*. New York: Random House, 1987.

Zinner, Stephen. *How to Protect Yourself from STDs*. New York: Summit Books, 1986.

MEDICAL

Broder, Samuel. *AIDS: Modern Concepts and Therapeutic Challenges*. New York: Marcel Dekker, 1986.

Brown, Raymond Keith. *AIDS, Cancer & The Medical Establishment*. New York: Robert Speller & Sons, 1986.

DeVita, Vincent T., Jr., Samuel Hellman, and Steven A. Rosenberg, eds. *AIDS: Etiology, Diagnosis, Treatment and Prevention*. Philadelphia: J. B. Lippincott Co., 1985.

Dunham, Jerry, and Felissa Lashley Cohen. *The Person With AIDS: Nursing Perspectives*. New York: Springer Publishing, 1987.

Ebbesen, Peter, Robert J. Biggar, and Made Malbye, eds. *AIDS: A Basic Guide For Clinicians*. Philadelphia: W.B. Saunders Co., 1984.

Flaskerud, Jacquelyn. *AIDS/HIV Infection: A Reference Guide for Nursing Professionals*. Philadelphia: W.B. Saunders Co., 1989.

Giraldo, G., and E. Beth, eds. *Epidemic of Acquired Immune Deficiency Syndrome (AIDS) and Kaposi's Sarcoma: Antibiotics and Chemotherapy*, Vol. 32. New York: S. Karger, 1984.

Hughes, Anne, Jeanne Parker Martin, and Pat Franks. *AIDS Home Care and Hospice Manual*. San Francisco: Visiting Nurses & Hospice of San Francisco, 1989.

Klein, Eva, ed. *Acquired Immunodeficiency Syndrome: Progress in Allergy*, Vol. 37. New York: S. Karger, 1986.

Kulstad, Ruth, ed. *AIDS: Papers from "Science" 1982-1985*. Boulder, Colo.: Westview Press, 1986.

Long, Robert Emmet. *AIDS: The Reference Shelf*, Vol. 59, Number 3. Bronx, N.Y.: H. W. Wilson, 1987.

Menitove, Jay E., and Jerry Kolins, eds. *AIDS*. Arlington, Va.: American Assoc. of Blood Banks, 1986.

Miller, David, Jonathan Weber, and John Green, eds. *The Management of AIDS Patients*. Dobbs Ferry, N.Y.: Sheridan House, 1985.

Nichols, Stuart E., and Daniel G. Ostrow, eds. *Psychiatric Implications of Acquired Immune Deficiency Syndrome*. Washington, D.C.: American Psychiatric Press, 1984.

Olweny, C. L. M., M. S. R. Hutt, and R. Owor, eds. *Kaposi's Sarcoma: Antibiotics and Chemotherapy*. New York: S. Karger, 1981.

Otter, Jean, ed. *The Current Status of HTLV-III Testing*. Arlington, Va.: American Assoc. of Blood Banks, 1986.

Petricciani, J. C., I. D. Gust, P. A. Hoppe, and H. W. Krijnen. *AIDS: The Safety of Blood and Blood Products*. New York: John Wiley & Sons, Inc., 1987.

Vaeth, J. M., ed. *Cancer and AIDS: Frontiers of Radiation Therapy and Oncology*, Vol 19. New York: S. Karger, 1985.

ALTERNATIVE HEALING/STRENGTHENING IMMUNE SYSTEM

Badgley, Laurence. *Healing AIDS Naturally*. San Bruno, Calif.: Human Energy Press, 1987.

Berger, Stuart. *Dr. Berger's Immune Power Diet*. New York: New American Library, 1985.

Kushi, Michio, and Martha Cottrell. *AIDS & Immune Deficiency: Macrobiotic Approach*. Japan Publications, 1987.

Muramoto, Noburu. *The AIDS-Related Diet: How the Food We Eat Builds or Destroys Immunity Against Infectious and Contagious Disease*. Oroville, Calif.: George Ohsawa Macrobiotic Foundation, 1988.

Russell-Manning, Betsy, ed. *Self-Treatment for AIDS: Oxygen Therapies*. Berkeley, Calif.: Celestial Arts, 1987.

Serinus, Jason, ed. *Psychoimmunity and the Healing Process: A Holistic Approach to Immunity and AIDS*. Berkeley, Calif.: Celestial Arts, 1986.

Tatchell, Peter. *AIDS: A Guide to Survival*. London: Gay Men's Press, 1986.

Weiner, Michael. *Maximum Immunity: How to Fortify Your Natural Defenses Against Cancer, AIDS, Arthritis, Allergies — Even the Common Cold — and Free Yourself from Unnecessary Worry for Life!* Boston: Houghton Mifflin Company, 1986.

PERSONAL STORIES/EMOTIONAL SUPPORT

Barbo, Beverly. *The Walking Wounded: A Mother's True Story of Her Son's Homosexuality and His Eventual AIDS Related Death*. Lindsborg, Kans.: Carlson's, 1987.

Hoyle, Jay. *Mark: How a Boy's Courage in Facing AIDS Inspired a Town and the Town's Compassion Lit Up a Nation*. South Bend, Ind.: Langford Books, 1988.

Hudson, Rock, and Sara Davidson. *Rock Hudson: His Story*. New York: Avon, 1987.

Moffatt, BettyClare. *When Someone You Love Has AIDS: A Book of Hope for Family and Friends*. New York: NAL/Plume, 1987.

Monette, Paul. *Borrowed Time*. San Diego, Calif.: Harcourt Brace Jovanovich, 1988.

Nungresser, Lou. *An Epidemic of Courage: Facing AIDS in America*. New York: St. Martin's Press, 1986.

Oyler, Chris. *Go Toward the Light: A Mother's Story—A Family's Love—A Child's Courage Facing Death*. New York: Harper & Row, 1988.

Peabody, Barbara. *The Screaming Room: A Mother's Journal of Her Son's Struggle With AIDS— A True Story of Love, Dedication, and Courage*. San Diego, Calif.: Oak Tree Publications, 1986.

Pearson, Carol Lynn. *Goodbye, I Love You: The True Story of a Wife, Her Homosexual Husband—and a Love Honored for Time and All Eternity*. New York: Random House, 1986.

Whitmore, George. *Someone Was Here: Profiles in the AIDS Epidemic*. New York: New American Library, 1988.

RELIGIOUS/SPIRITUAL

Amos, William, Jr. *When AIDS Comes to Church*. Philadelphia, Pa.: The Westminster Press, 1988.

The Catholic Health Association of the United States and The Conference of Major Religious Superiors of Men's Institutes of the United States. *The Gospel Alive: Caring for Persons With AIDS and Related Illnesses*. St. Louis, Mo.: The Catholic Health Assoc., 1988.

Flynn, Eileen. *AIDS: A Catholic Call for Compassion*. Kansas City, Mo.: Sheed & Ward, 1986.

Fortunato, John. *AIDS: The Spiritual Dilemma*. New York: Harper & Row, 1987.

Shelp, Earl, and Ronald Sunderland. *AIDS and the Church*. Louisville, Ky.: Westminster Press, 1987.

Shelp, Earl, Ronald Sunderland, and Peter Mansell. *AIDS: Personal Stories in Pastoral Perspective*. New York: Pilgrim Press, 1986.

Tinney, James. *Pastoral Care for the Person With AIDS*. Washington, D.C.: Faith Temple, 1985.

Tuohey, John. *Caring for Persons with AIDS and Cancer: Ethical Reflections on Palliative Care for the Terminally Ill*. St. Louis, Mo.: The Catholic Health Assoc., 1988.

DEATH & DYING/GRIEF RECOVERY

Moffatt, BettyClare. *Gifts for the Living: Conversations with Caregivers on Death and Dying*. Santa Monica, Calif.: IBS Press, 1988.

Parrish-Harra, Carol. *The New Age Handbook On Death and Dying*. Santa Monica, Calif.: IBS Press, 1989.

Roth, Deborah, *Being Human in the Face of Death*. Santa Monica, Calif.: IBS Press, 1989.

Roth, Deborah. *Stepping Stones to Grief Recovery*. Santa Monica, Calif.: IBS Press, 1987.

WOMEN

Norwood, Chris. *Advice for Life: A Woman's Guide to AIDS Risks and Prevention*. New York: Pantheon, 1987.

Patton, Cindy, and Janice Kelly. *Making It: A Woman's Guide to Sex in the Age of AIDS*. Ithaca, N.Y.: Firebrand Books, 1987.

Richardson, Diane. *Women & AIDS*. New York: Methuen, 1988.

Rieder, Ines, and Patricia Ruppelt. *AIDS: The Women*. Pittsburgh, Pa.: Cleis Press, 1988.

LEGAL

Dalton, Harlan, and Scott Burris. *AIDS and the Law: A Guide for the Public*. New Haven, Conn.: Yale University Press, 1987.

Dornette, William. *AIDS and the Law*. New York: John Wiley & Sons, 1987.

FICTION

Bryan, Jed. *A Cry in the Desert*. Austin, Tex.: Banned Books, 1987.

Ferro, Robert. *Second Son*. New York: Crown, 1988.

Fierstein, Harvey. *Safe Sex*. New York: Atheneum, 1987.

Hoffman, Alice. *At Risk*. New York: G. P. Putnam's Sons, 1988.

Monette, Paul. *Love Alone: Eighteen Elegies for Rog*. New York: St. Martin's Press, 1988.

Reed, Paul. *Facing It: A Novel of AIDS*. San Francisco: Gay Sunshine Press, 1984.

Warmbold, Jean. *June Mail*. Sag Harbor, N.Y.: The Permanent Press, 1986.

BOOKS FOR YOUNGER READERS

de Saint Phalle, Niki. *AIDS: You Can't Catch It Holding Hands*. San Francisco: The Lapis Press, 1987.

Hyde, Margaret, and Elizabeth Forsyth. *AIDS: What Does It Mean to You?* New York: Walker & Co., 1987.

Hyde, Margaret, and Elizabeth Forsyth. *Know About AIDS*. New York: Walker & Co., 1987.

Kerr, M. E. *Night Kites*. New York: Harper & Row, 1986.

Lerner, Ethan. *Understanding AIDS*. Minneapolis, Minn.: Lerner Publications, 1987. (612)232-3344.

Marsh, Carole. *Sex Stuff: A Book of Practical Information & Ideas for Kids 7-17, and Their Teachers and Parents*. Bath, N.C.: Gallopade Publishing Group, 1987.

Miklowitz, Gloria. *Good-Bye Tomorrow*. New York: Delacorte Press, 1987.

Nourse, Alan. *AIDS*. New York: Franklin Watts, 1986.

Wachter, Oralee. *Sex, Drugs and AIDS*. New York: Bantam, 1987.

Young, Alida. *I Never Got to say Good-Bye*. Worthington, Ohio: Willowisp Press, 1988.

BOOKS FOR PARENTS AND TEACHERS

Kaus, Danek, and Robert Reed. *AIDS, Your Child and the School*. Saratoga, Calif.: R & E Research Associates, 1986.

Kaus, Danek, and Robert Reed. *Teaching About AIDS*. Saratoga, Calif.: R & E Research Associates, 1987.

Weisman, Betsy, and Michael Weisman. *What We Told Our Kids About Sex*. San Diego, Calif.: Harcourt Brace Jovanovich/Harvest, 1987.

BIBLIOGRAPHIC REFERENCES /DIRECTORIES

AIDS Bibliography. GPO ID: AID88. Order from U.S. Government Printing Office, Washington, DC 20402. (202)783-3238.

AIDS 1988: Oryx Science Bibliography. Phoenix, Ariz.: Oryx Press, 1988.

AIDS: A Bibliography. Saratoga, Calif.: R & E Publishers, 1987.

The AIDS Catalog. Saratoga, Calif.: R & E Publishers, 1988.

AIDS Data Base Directory. Medical Data Exchange, 445 South San Antonio Rd., Los Altos, CA 94019. (415)941-3600.

AIDS: How & Where to Find Facts and Do Research. Saratoga, Calif.: R & E Publishers, 1987.

AIDS Information Resources Directory. American Foundation for AIDS Research, 1515 Broadway #3601, New York, NY 10036. Order from R.R. Bowker, 1-800-521-8110.

The AIDS Information Sourcebook. Phoenix, Ariz.: Oryx Press, 1988.

AIDS Literature & News Review. University Publishing Group, 107 East Church St., Frederick, MD 21701.

AIDS: Law Ethics & Public Policy. (Bibliography). Order from Scope Note Series, Kennedy Institute of Ethics, Georgetown University, Poullon Hall 210, Washington, DC 20057. 1-800-MED-ETHX.

The AIDS Record Directory of Key AIDS Program Officials in Federal, State, County and City Governments. Bio-Data Publishers, P.O. Box 66020, Washington, DC 20035. (202)393-AIDS.

AIDS Reference and Research Collection. University Publishing Group, 107 East Church St., Frederick, MD 21701.

AIDS Service Directory for Hispanics. National Coalition of Hispanic Health & Human Services Organizations, 1030 15th St. NW, Suite 1053, Washington, DC 20005. (202)371-2100.

Computerized AIDS Information Network. 1213 N. Highland Ave., Los Angeles, CA 90038. (213)464-7400, ext. 277.

Directory of AIDS Related Services. United States Conference of Mayors, 1620 "I" St. NW, Washington, DC 20006. (202)293-7330.

Educating About AIDS. (Catalog). Network Publications/ETR Associates, P.O. Box 1830, Santa Cruz, CA 95061. (408)438-4080.

Hero Catalog. Hero, Inc., 101 West Read St., Baltimore, MD 21201.
(301)685-1180.

National Library of Medicine Literature Search - AIDS Series. National
Library of Medicine, 8600 Rockville Pike, Bethesda, MD 20894.
(301)496-6095.

PERIODICALS

AIDS Alert. American Health Consultants, Department 4651,
67 Peachtree Park Dr. N.E., Atlanta, GA 30309.

AIDSFILE. San Francisco General Hospital, Ward 84,
1001 Portrero St., San Francisco, CA 94110. (415)821-5531.

AIDS Information Exchange. United States Conference of Mayors,
1620 Eye St. N.W., Washington, DC 20006.

AIDS Law & Litigation Reporter. University Publishing Group,
107 East Church St., Frederick, MD 21701.

AIDS Medical Update. UCLA, 12-248 Factor Bldg.,
Los Angeles, CA 90024. (213)825-1510.

AIDS Nursing Update. UCLA, 12-248 Factor Bldg.,
Los Angeles, CA 90024. (213)825-1510.

AIDS Policy & Law Newsletter. Buraff Publications,
2445 "M" St. N.W., Suite 275, Washington, DC 20037.

AIDS Protection. National AIDS Prevention Institute,
205 South East St., Culpepper, VA 22701. (701)825-4040.

AIDS & Public Policy Journal. University Publishing Group,
107 East Church St., Frederick, MD 21701.

The AIDS Record. Bio-Data Publishers,
P.O. Box 66020, Washington, DC 20035.

AIDS Targeted Information Newsletter. Williams & Wilkins,
428 E. Preston St., Baltimore, MD 21202. 1-800-638-6423.

AIDS Update. Santa Barbara County Health Care,
300 N. San Antonio Rd., Santa Barbara, CA 93110. (805)681-5120.

AIDS Weekly Surveillance Report. Centers for Disease Control,
1360 Peachtree St., Atlanta, GA 30309. (404)329-5138.

ALERT. Universal Fellowship of Metropolitan Community Churches,
5300 Santa Monica Blvd., Suite 304, Los Angeles, CA 90029. (213)464-5100.

CDC AIDS Weekly. CDC, P.O. Box 5528, Atlanta, GA 30307

FDA Talk Paper - Update On Experimental AIDS Therapies and Vaccines.
FDA, 5600 Fisher's Lane, Room 1505, Rockville, MD 20857. (301)443-3285.

FOCUS: A Guide to AIDS Research & Counseling. AIDS Health Project,
Box 0884, San Francisco, CA 94143. (415)476-6430.

NAPWA News. National Association of PWA,
2025 "I" St. NW, Suite 415, Washington, DC 20006. (202)429-2856.

Network News. National AIDS Network,
1012 14th St. NW, Suite 601, Washington, DC 20005. (202)347-0390.

Surviving & Thriving with AIDS: Hints for the Newly Diagnosed.
PWA Coalition, 222 West 11th, New York, NY 10011. (212)627-1810.

MEDICAL JOURNALS:
These journals often carry breaking news on AIDS.

Annals of Internal Medicine

Journal of the American Medical Association

The Lancet

Morbidity & Mortality Weekly Report. Order from U.S. Government
Printing Office, Washington, DC 20402. (202)783-3238.

New England Journal of Medicine

Science

GAY/LESBIAN PRESS:
These periodicals report regularly on the AIDS epidemic and related issues.

The Advocate, The New York Native (National)

The Bay Area Reporter, Coming Up!, The Sentinel (San Francisco)

Gay Community News (Boston)

Philadelphia Gay News

Washington Blade

AUDIO TAPES

AIDS and Anger. Sally Fisher. Order from W.A.S.H. Productions, 952 N. Orange Grove, Los Angeles, CA 90046.

Living Powerfully with AIDS. Sally Fisher. Order from W.A.S.H. Productions, 952 N. Orange Grove, Los Angeles, CA 90046.

Overcoming AIDS: Hypno-Sleep Tape. Seth Hermes Foundation, P.O. Box 4111, Simi Valley, CA 93063.

Overcoming AIDS: Subliminal Motivation. Seth Hermes Foundation, P.O. Box 4111, Simi Valley, CA 93063.

Relaxation and Visualization. AIDS Health Project, Box 0884, San Francisco, CA 94143.

Sixty Minutes to Smart Sex. Dr. Dean Edell. Available from Audio Renaissance Tapes, 9110 Sunset Blvd. #240, Los Angeles, CA 90069.

Self-care Data Flow Sheet

DATE				
TIME				
TEMPERATURE				
SYMPTOMS: Sweats (Y,N)				
Chills (Y,N)				
Fatigue (Y,N)				
WEIGHT				
MEDICATIONS: (Name, dose, time taken)				
FLUID INTAKE (type, amt., & time)				
URINE OUTPUT (time & amt. - S, M, L)				
DIARRHEA (time & amt. S,M,L)				
FOOD INTAKE Breakfast				
Lunch				
Dinner				
Snacks				
COMMENTS: (other symptoms, visits to Dr., treatments, etc.)				

Summary of Your Health Coverage

Your Full Name _____

Your Address _____

_____

Employer's Name _____

Address _____

_____

Tel. Number _____

Insurance Co. Name _____

Claims Address _____

Your Policy / ID Number _____

Your Contact at Claims Office _____

Maximum Benefit _____   Deductible _____

Co-Insurance _____   Stop-Loss Point _____

Hospital Rm & Bd Rates _____   # Days Limitations _____

Intensive Care Rates _____

Special Features / LImitations _____

_____

_____

Psychological Benefits _____

Limitations _____

Insurance Co. Home Office Address _____

_____

Getting Your Affairs in Order

Your Name _____

*Address:*_____

_____

*Telephone:*_____

Social Security Number: _____

Birthdate: _____

IN CASE OF EMERGENCY CONTACT

Name: _____

Address:_____

_____

Telephone: (h) _____ (w) _____

Nearest Relative:

Name: _____

Telephone (h) _____ (w) _____

RESOURCE CONTACTS

Employer:_____

Telephone: _____

Doctor(s):_____

Telephone: _____

Attorney: _____

_____

Telephone: _____

Accountant/Bookeeper: _____

_____

Telephone: _____

FINANCIAL

Checking account

Bank: _____

Branch: _____

Acct. #: _____

Savings account

Bank: _____

Branch: _____

Acct. #: _____

Credit union

Branch: _____

Acct. #: _____

Other

Certificates: _____

_____

Stocks, bonds: _____

_____

Retirement Accts.: _____

_____

_____

Real Estate: _____

_____

How title is held: _____

Loans to others: _____

_____

Reprinted with permission from a brochure of the San Francisco AIDS Foundation, in cooperation with the Bay Area Lawyers for Individual Freedom.

Deficits

Loans:

Mortagage: _____

_____

Car loan: _____

Personal: _____

_____

Other: _____

_____

_____

_____

CREDIT ACCOUNTS/CARDS

VISA/Mastercharge/other:

_____ # _____

_____ # _____

_____ # _____

_____ # _____

_____ # _____

Dept. stores/gas cards:

_____ # _____

_____ # _____

_____ # _____

_____ # _____

_____ # _____

_____ # _____

_____ # _____

_____ # _____

INSURANCE COVERAGE

Health Insurance

Name of Company: _____

Address: _____

Telephone: _____

Agent/contact: _____

Life Insurance

Name of Company: _____

Address: _____

Telephone: _____

Agent/contact: _____

Disability Insurance

Name of Company: _____

Address: _____

Telephone: _____

Agent/contact: _____

Auto/Home/Other Insurance

Name of Company: _____

Address: _____

Telephone: _____

Agent/contact: _____

Name of Company: _____

Address: _____

Telephone: _____

Agent/contact: _____

DOCUMENTS

Will

Location: _____

Date: _____

Rental/Lease Agreement

Location: _____

Deposits to be returned: _____

_____

Tax Records

Location: _____

_____

Real Estate Documents

Location: _____

_____

Safe Deposit Box

Location: _____

_____

Location of key: _____

Who has access to box: _____

_____

Vehicle Registration: # _____

Location of forms: _____

Vehicle License: # _____

Other Documents: _____

_____

MISCELLANEOUS

Possessions to be listed in your will that you would like individuals to receive:

Item   **Person's Name**

_____

_____

_____

_____

_____

_____

_____

_____

_____

_____

_____

Who has copies of this form?

_____

_____

_____

_____

_____

_____

_____

_____

Tracking Your Insurance Claims

	Dates of Service	Description of Service And Dates of Service	Provider of Service	Date Sent to Ins.Co.	I Paid	Date	Ins.Co Paid	Balance Due
1.								
2.								
3.								
4.								
5.								
6.								
7.								
8.								
9.								
10.								
11.								
12.								
13.								
14.								
15.								
16.								
17.								
18.								
19.								
20.								

	Balance Due	Payment on Balance Due #1	#2	#3	#4	#5	Date Fully Paid Off	Comments Follow-up Date Notes
1.								
2.								
3.								
4.								
5.								
6.								
7.								
8.								
9.								
10.								
11.								
12.								
13.								
14.								
15.								
16.								
17.								
18.								
19.								
20.								

List of Contributors

The following people contributed information to *AIDS: A Self-Care Manual:*

Donald Abrams, M.D.
Assistant Director, AIDS Clinic
Assistant Clinical Professor of Medicine
University of California San Francisco

John Acevedo, M.S.W.
Clinical Social Worker, AIDS Health
  Project,
University of California San Francisco

Rev. Brad Andersson

Walter Batchelor
Research Associate
Center for Applied Social Science
Boston University

Cherrie B. Boyer, Ph.D.
University of California San Francisco

Frank Carussi

Kenneth Charles

Chelsea Psychotherapy Group
  Michael Shernoff, C.S.W., A.C.S.W.
  Dixie Beckham, C.S.W., A.C.S.W.
  Vincent Pattie, C.S.W., A.C.S.W.
  Luis Palacios-Jimenez, C.S.W.,
    A.C.S.W.

Rev. Wayne Christiansen
Spiritual Advisory Committee
AIDS Project Los Angeles

Ralph J. DiClemente, Ph.D.
University of California San Francisco

Shelby Dietrich, M.D.
Director
Hemophilia Center at the Orthopedic
  Hospital, Los Angeles

David Epstein, Ph.D.

Chuck Frutchey
AIDS Hotline Coordinator, San Francisco
  AIDS Foundation

Jim Geary
Executive Director, Shanti, San Franciso.

Jaak Hamilton, M.A., M.F.C.C.
Board of Directors, AIDS Project Los
  Angeles

Graeme Hanson, M.D.
Director, Pediatric Mental Health Services
San Francisco General Hospital

Michael Helquist
Editor, *FOCUS: A Review of AIDS
  Research*
Editor, *Working with AIDS: A Resource
  Guide for Mental Health Professionals*
Columnist, *The Helquist Report,
  The Advocate*

Coleen Johnson, M.S.W.

Robert Krasnow, M.D.
Director, VA Hospital Hospice Program

Jennifer Lang, R.N., M.N.
Oncology Clinical Nurse Specialist

Rev. Bill Leeson
Spiritual Advisory Committee
AIDS Project Los Angeles

Ronald Mitsuyasu, M.D.
Assistant Professor of Medicine
Division of Hematology-Oncology, UCLA
  Medical Center

Alan Malyon, Ph.D.

BettyClare Moffatt, M.A.,
Author, *When Someone You Love Has
  AIDS: A Book of Hope for Family and
  Friends,* April 1986, IBS Press; April
  1987, New American Library
Co-founder MAP (Mothers of AIDS
  Patients) Los Angeles Chapter

Stephen Morin, Ph.D.
Assistant Clinical Professor of Medicine,
    UCSF
Clinical Psychologist in Private Practice

Brent Nance, CLU
Insurance Counselor, AIDS Project Los
    Angeles

Buck Nunes
Staff Member, San Francisco
    AIDS Foundation

Tristano Palermino
Former Director of Social Services
San Francisco AIDS Foundation

Allan Pinka, Ph.D.

Rev. Steve Pieters
Board Member, AIDS Project Los Angeles

Rev. Stephen D. Preston
Spiritual Advisory Committee
AIDS Project Los Angeles

Marcia Quackenbush, M.S., M.F.C.C.
Coordinator of the Youth and
    AIDS Prevention Program
UCSF AIDS Health Project
Co-author, *Teaching AIDS: A Resource
    Guide on AIDS*

Richard Rector
Co-chair, National People with
    AIDS Association
Administrative Assistant, AIDS Activity
    Office
San Mateo County

Rex Reece, Ph.D.
Coordinator, Education Subcommittee,
    Psychosocial Advisory Council and
    Member, Board of Directors, AIDS
    Project Los Angeles

Rev. Tom Reinhart-Marean

Robert Reynolds
Co-director, National Association of People
    with AIDS;
Board Member, Shanti Project, San
    Francisco

Andrew Rose, M.S.W., L.C.S.W

Nancy Stoller Shaw, Ph.D.
Coordinator of Women's Programs
San Francisco AIDS Foundation

Scott Sherman, Ph.D.
Didi Hirsch Community Mental Health
    Center

Neil Schram, M.D.
Chair, Mayor's City/County AIDS Task
    Force

Judith A. Spiegel, M.P.H.
Director of Information and Education.
AIDS Project Los Angeles

Stephen M. Strigle, B.S., C.T. (ACSP)
Assistant Instructor
School of Cytotechnology, Los Angeles
    County–USC
Medical Center Chair

Roslyn Sussman, L.C.S.W.
Clinical AIDS Specialist/Hemophilia
Orthopedic Hospital, Los Angeles

Roberta J. Wong, Pharm.D.
Clinical Research Pharmacist
San Francisco General Hospital

John Ziegler, M.D.
Director, AIDS Clinical Research Center

INDEX

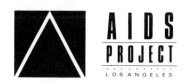

AIDS PROJECT
LOS ANGELES

This self-care manual is just one example of the work of AIDS Project Los Angeles. AIDS Project Los Angeles is a non-profit organization dedicated to improving the quality of life for persons with AIDS and ARC and their loved ones.

Your gift helps fulfill their needs of food, shelter, dental care and counseling, and enables AIDS Project Los Angeles to share the facts about AIDS with the general public. For now, education is our only hope to stop the spread of AIDS.

To join the fight against AIDS, send this reply card with your donation to:

AIDS Project Los Angeles
6721 Romaine Street
West Hollywood, CA 90038

I would like to share this information with others ...

QUANTITY	BOOK TITLES	PRICE	TOTAL
	AIDS: A SELF-CARE MANUAL, 3rd Edition -- *AIDS Project Los Angeles*	$14.95	
	WHEN SOMEONE YOU LOVE HAS AIDS: A Book of Hope for Family and Friends -- *BettyClare Moffatt, M.A.*	8.95	
	GIFTS FOR THE LIVING: Conversations with Caregivers on Death and Dying -- *BettyClare Moffatt, M.A.*	9.95	
	STEPPING STONES TO GRIEF RECOVERY -- *Deborah Roth, M.S.C.*	8.95	
	THE NEW AGE HANDBOOK ON DEATH AND DYING -- *Rev.Carol W. Parrish-Harra*	9.95	
	BEING HUMAN IN THE FACE OF DEATH--*Deborah Roth & Emily LeVier*	9.95	
	SURVIVORS OF SUICIDE -- *Rita Robinson*	9.95	
	THE LAW OF MIND IN ACTION -- *Dr. Fenwicke Lindsay Holmes*	10.95	
	SHIPPING & HANDLING ($2.00 per book)		
	Sales Tax 6.5% (California residents only)		
	TOTAL DUE		

Please send check or money order to:
IBS PRESS, 744 Pier Avenue, Santa Monica, CA 90405 (213)450-6485

Name _____

Address _____

City/State/Zip _____

Quantity Discounts are Available to AIDS-Related Organizations

AIDS Project Los Angeles
6721 Romaine Street
West Hollywood, CA 90038

IBS Press
744 Pier Avenue
Santa Monica, CA 90405